Atlas of Canine Surgical Techniques

EDITED BY

P. G. C. BEDFORD

BVetMed, PhD, FRCVS, DV Ophthal
Royal Veterinary College Field Station
North Mymms, Hatfield
Hertfordshire

FOR THE

British Small Animal
Veterinary Association

BLACKWELL SCIENTIFIC PUBLICATIONS

OXFORD LONDON EDINBURGH

BOSTON PALO ALTO MELBOURNE

TO TEA, VICTORIA AND
NICHOLAS
whose contribution was
immeasurable

© 1984 by
Blackwell Scientific Publications
Editorial offices:
Osney Mead, Oxford, OX2 0EL
8 John Street, London, WC1N 2ES
9 Forrest Road, Edinburgh, EH1 2QH
52 Beacon Street, Boston
    Massachusetts 02108, USA
706 Cowper Street, Palo Alto
    California 94301, USA
99 Barry Street, Carlton
    Victoria 3053, Australia

First published 1984

Photoset by Enset Ltd.
Midsomer Norton, Bath, Avon
and printed and bound by
The Camelot Press Ltd, Southampton

DISTRIBUTORS

USA
    Blackwell Mosby Book Distributors
    11830 Westline Industrial Drive
    St Louis, Missouri 63141

Canada
    Blackwell Mosby Book Distributors
    120 Melford Drive, Scarborough
    Ontario, M1B 2X4

Australia
    Blackwell Scientific Book Distributors
    31 Advantage Road, Highett
    Victoria 3190

British Library
Cataloguing in Publication Data

Atlas of canine surgical techniques.
    1. Dogs — Surgery
    I. Bedford, P.G.C.
    636.7′0897   SF991

ISBN 0-632-01154-8

Contents

Preface

The relatively recent and ongoing expansion of small animal veterinary medicine in the UK has led quite naturally to increased interest in the development of surgical treatments. This development for the dog has been a rapid one with new techniques making their appearance in the literature with impressive regularity. Time and the availability of specialized equipment would appear to be the only limiting factors involved in the extent of canine surgery possible within practice, and obviously balance must be maintained between the volume of routine clinical work attempted and the extent of the surgical service provided. Once the factors of time and equipment have been resolved, and given interest and dexterity, then it is a working knowledge of surgical anatomy and technique that builds towards experience and, with that, success. It is with these objectives in mind that this textbook has been compiled, the basic premise employed being the investigation of the extent of canine surgery that could be possible within the average small animal practice. Thus the authors are clinicians primarily involved in referral work, and they have selected the type of surgery that they are routinely asked to perform which could be done successfully from a practice base given some further practical advice on technique and equipment. With this specific remit in view, this textbook does not set out to be a compendium of surgery for the dog. Routine surgical techniques have not been included, and neither have those techniques which would be rarely performed within any one practice and which would require extensive specialized instrumentation. Rather it is the 'middle-ground' which is explored, and though the techniques included are neither original nor exhaustive, in the authors' opinion they jointly represent a practical attempt towards the improvement of the surgical service generally available within practice. Clinical evaluation of the patient and diagnosis have been largely assumed, but it was considered that practical advice on radiography, anaesthesia and fluid therapy should be included in a textbook of this nature.

Acknowledgements

This publication could never have taken form without the generous assistance of the several authors involved. My thanks go to them for their adherence to my guidelines and the overall excellence of their contributions. Particular thanks go to Jennie Smith for her enthusiastic approach in producing the many superb illustrations contained within the atlas section of the book.

Section 1
Surgical Instrumentation, Anaesthesia, Fluid Therapy and Radiography

Part A
Surgical Instrumentation

GORDON J. BAKER

Introduction

The primary goal of the surgical treatment of disease, i.e. its cure, the relief of pain and the restoration of function, is achieved by manipulative, incisive, excisive or plastic means. The surgeon should keep in mind that whatever process is used, it will be both traumatic and stressful. The successful outcome of the procedure depends upon the optimum use of the equipment and the environment and it must be emphasized that the three basic rules of surgery are cleanliness, efficiency (that includes speed), and gentleness. The most frequently encountered surgical faults result from a breakdown of these rules, i.e. there is contamination and/or protracted surgical time and/or tissue trauma. The good surgeon is one who applies the skills of manipulation, incision, excision or repair in a manner so constructed that the best results are achieved within the minimum of trauma and the minimum of stress. The old adage that a bad workman blames his tools is true; what may be more pertinent, however, is that the truly bad surgeon doesn't even know that the tools and techniques are bad!

Surgical instruments should be selected to suit the purpose for which they are to be used, and conversely that means that every instrument must only be used for its designed purpose. We are all too well aware of surgical equipment being forced to undertake tasks for which it was not designed, e.g. the use of needle holders or artery forceps to extract Steinmann pins after fracture fixation. This may well work in that the pin will be extracted, but the price will be strained joints or box locks and damaged jaws on the forceps. The cost of surgical instruments may appear to be extraordinarily high, but it is worth noting that the high quality will normally more than repay the investment. The use of tungsten carbide inserts in the blades of scissors and the jaws of needle holders is to be recommended.

The basic surgical set consists of instruments for cutting, dissection, instruments for grasping, retraction, haemostasis and ligating, and suturing. In the past 10 or 15 years there have been considerable developments in the production of more elegant surgical equipment, and a brief perusal of any reputable manufacturing company's catalogue will give the prospective buyer a plethora of instruments from which to choose. Quite commonly many instruments have often been designed by particular surgeons and therefore retain their names, e.g. Metzenbaum thyroid scissors. We have seen major developments in the production of new lighting facilities, more efficient diathermy and suction equipment and of microsurgical equipment and operating microscopes. As far as orthopaedic surgery is concerned, major developments stem from the equipment developed by the Arbeitsgemeinschaft für Osteosynthesefragen (AO or Association for the Study of Problems of Internal Fixation, ASIF). Similar equipment is available from a number of instrument manufacturers and is widely used in small animal orthopaedic surgery.

The clinician must also be aware that specific developments in the veterinary field have only been possible thanks to the coordinated efforts of other specialized fields. Nowadays, advanced surgical techniques should be performed by a team of 'specialists' thereby meeting the fourth rule of surgery, i.e. the finest results are achieved by the summation of the skills of the team of specialists. In our case the anaesthetist, clinical pathologist, nursing staff and surgical assistants are all important.

Clinicians are advised to consult with the referral hospitals and to visit instrument retailers so that a personal touch can be gained. The surgeon should get a good feeling from handling any prospective purchase; this assumes certain manual confidence and dexterities that only practice can achieve. In this manner, the best equipment will be obtained, it will be used *correctly* and, more importantly, the best results will be achieved. As the old saying goes 'some people make the same mistakes a hundred times and call it experience' (Mayo), and that is not the experience we are trying to achieve.

Surgical instruments

Scalpels

The scalpel is the basic cutting instrument of the surgeon. The Bard–Parker is the prototype of the scalpel design in which disposable scalpel blades are used and a range of scalpel blade and handle sizes and shapes are available. The scalpel should be drawn across tissues rather than driven into them, a single long stroke being less traumatic and more effective than multiple small cuts. Using a No. 10 blade, the scalpel should be used at an angle of 30–40° to the skin. There are two acceptable and convenient styles for handling the scalpel. It may be grasped by the thumb and middle finger so that the handle rests in the palm and the index finger is then placed on top of the instrument for stability. It can also be used in the pencil grip when angling the blade at 30–40° may endanger surrounding tissues. The blade should be loaded and removed using a needle holder, not with the fingers.

Scissors

Scissors are classified and identified by their length, shape, blade tip form and their use. Blade tip may be blunt on blunt, blunt on sharp or sharp on sharp. As mentioned earlier, care should be taken to ensure that the correct instrument is used for the right purpose. Tissue dissecting and cutting scissors should not be used to cut, suture or ligature material or wire. In the basic surgical set and for most surgical purposes, straight and curved 6-inch Mayo scissors, together with an 8-inch Metzenbaum dissection scissors can be used for most purposes. In addition, a straight blunt/sharp tipped suture scissors is included.

Blunt dissection is achieved by inserting the points and opening the handles, maintaining the hand in pronation. By keeping the thumb and finger rings near the ends of the fingers rather than allowing the rings to slide up the fingers, greater range of movement in dissection and manipulation can be achieved. When scissors are used for cutting tissue, the surgeon is reminded that the scissor blade is basically a crushing instrument. Consequently, a greater accuracy and the less traumatic incision is made if the scissors are used as a slicing instrument rather than a chopping instrument. To achieve this the blade is inserted, elevated and then the scissor is simply pushed through the tissue.

Forceps

This group of instruments shows a range both in shape and purpose. It is convenient to describe the forceps based on their function, dressing and tissue forceps. Dressing or thumb forceps consist of two tines or blades connected at one end, aligned so as to spring open. The tips may be smooth or have teeth (rat's tooth). Smooth forceps, e.g. Ewald, may be used to handle vessels or intestine. Large toothed forceps should only be used for dense tissue. The most common compromise between the smooth and toothed is the Brown–Adson forceps. Such a thumb forceps is the most satisfactory instrument for handling tissue during dissection, excision, or during suture procedures. The instrument is held in the assisting hand of the operator and instrument is held in the assisting hand of the operator and should be held like a pencil so that the greatest range of movement can be gained. The anatomy dissection room technique of the heavy grip with the instrument held in the palm should be discouraged.

Haemostatic forceps

These instruments are used to hold and clamp vessels. They range in size from 3–9 inches; they usually have a box lock joint, and they vary primarily in the size and shape of their tips. The mosquito is the smallest forceps that will afford haemostasis. It should be remembered that the more tissue that is grasped in any forceps the greater will be the surgical trauma. Therefore, grasp the tissue with only the tips of the forceps. Haemostasis may be obtained by forcipressure alone or by ligation around the forceps or by coagulation down the forceps using the diathermy. Larger vessels should be divided between forceps. A wide range of tip design and forceps shape is available. Spencer–Wells and Rochester–Péan forceps have transverse grooves throughout their length and are useful for the control of large vessels or tissue bundles. Kelly forceps are only grooved on their tips and so should not be used other than for fine vessels. Carmalts and Rochester–Carmalts have longitudinal grooves and facilitate ligation. Specialized haemostatic forceps, the angiotribe, and such vascular forceps as the Satinsky, Dieffenbach bulldog clips all have their role in specific operations. Cardiovascular forceps, e.g. the

DeBakey range, incorporate the patented Kapp–Beck rounded serrations that give 100% occlusion with minimal trauma.

Tissue forceps

These are designed specifically for holding tissue. The Allis tissue forceps is designed to produce minimum tissue trauma with maximum holding power, but should be used on dense tissue only, not skin and bowel. The Babcock tissue forceps is of similar design to the Allis, but does not have interlocking jaws. Further jaw modifications are made in Duval lung holders and Vulsellum tissue forceps to both decrease and increase grasping strength. Towel clamps or forceps are used to secure skin drapes and are placed at 45° across the corner of two drapes. Various patterns are available; the Backhaus clamp is suitable for most situations. After application, the handles are tucked beneath the drape so as to leave an unobstructed surface, and avoid exposed suture or ligature material becoming entangled with the clamp.

Bowel forceps

These are available in a variety of sizes and designs. The Babcock tissue forceps can be used to handle bowel and contents can be controlled by application of forceps across the lumen. However, forceps with longitudinal serrations are preferred to facilitate their removal after stump closure. The large Rochester–Péan forceps are used when the stump is to be crushed and inverted, whilst the Doyen bowel forceps have a softer grip (fewer grooves) and may be used with rubber sleeves to control bowel content with the minimum of trauma to the viscus.

Needle holders

Most needle holders resemble haemostatic forceps with modification of the tips and the handles. The handles are shorter and heavier and have crossed grooving. Tips with tungsten carbide inserts prolong the life and give a more secure grip on the needle shaft. Needle holders may be long or short and may incorporate a ratchet locking device on the handle or a scissor blade. The Mayo–Hegar or Metzenbaum are widely used. The forceps should be 'palmed' with the tip of the thumb through one ring, and in this manner the needle is placed through tissue with a rolling action of the wrist.

Retractors

These are used to facilitate the exposure of the surgical field with minimal trauma and may be held by the surgical assistant or they may be self-retaining. Again, many types and patterns are available to the surgeon and they are an invaluable asset. This might be the point to confirm that the most useful surgical instruments available are another pair of skilled hands, with retractor attached! Useful retractors include the Senn, Parker, Langenbeck and the Hohmann. Malleable (copper) retractors come in various blade widths and may be bent by the surgeon to fit the particular circumstances. Self-retaining retractors are held open by a box lock or spring. Two commonly used examples are the Gelpi muscle retractor and the Weitlaner mastoid retractor. In thoracic surgery a stronger retractor is required with blunt tips, and one that usually incorporates a rib-spreading device, e.g. the Finochietto.

Electrocautery and suction

Both of these pieces of equipment are invaluable in aiding with haemostasis and by so doing improve the surgeon's visibility. Two basic types of electrocautery are available; the unipolar and the bipolar systems. As with forceps haemostasis, small vessels can be sealed completely but larger vessels will still require ligation. Recent developments have introduced the electric scalpel and the laser knife.

Effective wound irrigation is made possible by good wound aspiration and is recommended in all major surgical procedures.

Orthopaedic equipment

Major orthopaedic instruments are available in two metal alloys—stainless steel and vitallium. The latter is the most inert. It has been stated many times that mixed metals must not be used. This may be clear when plates and screws or pins and wires are concerned, but it is also true when instruments, drills, screwdrivers, etc., are used. Great care must therefore be taken in setting up the orthopaedic set so that it is compatible with the general surgery set.

ASIF equipment (Figs 4, 5 and 6) meets all of these requirements. Such equipment incorporates advanced plate, pin, and screw design as well as compressed air power tools.

Ophthalmic equipment

The refinement in this instance is related to the small size of the instruments involved, and misuse during surgery together with insufficient care between operations can result in reduced usefulness over a very short period of time. The basic set should include a versatile rat-tooth dressing forceps, e.g. St Martin's, and spring-handled needle holders, e.g. Castroviejo. Small scissors, e.g. Pooley's conjunctival scissors, and a 'tangle-free' speculum, e.g. Barraquer, are also essential (Fig. 8).

Drapes

For many procedures, disposable drapes or single fenestrated drapes may be used. Care must be taken, however, to ensure that at all times the patient is completely covered. All too often improper patient preparation and incomplete draping results in serious contamination of the surgical site. In some cases layered draping is essential. Following four corner draping and incision, the wound edges may be redraped or 'towelled in' and wound protectors (plastic and impervious) may be applied. In the author's hands, adhesive drapes have been singularly ineffective in veterinary surgery.

Limbs may be completely closed inside rolled stockingette drapes for orthopaedic procedures.

Care and maintenance

A number of surgical manufacturers offer an instrument maintenance and repair contract system and it is to be recommended if the best use is to be made of top price equipment. If care is taken in their maintenance, their sterilization, their packing and their handling, then quality instruments should outlive the surgeon.

After use, the instruments should be divided so that heavy pieces, chisels and other orthopaedic equipment are separated from the smaller, more delicate pieces. Scalpel blades should be removed and disposed of. All blood, tissue debris and materials should be cleansed immediately. Instruments should be washed in warm water with a mild detergent, keeping the ratchets and the box locks open. Once washed they may then be dried and resterilized. The use of ultrasonic cleansers requires proper instrument loading and additional care. Their use is an adjunct to, and not a replacement for, the initial washing procedure. Once the instruments have been dried they should be repacked carefully in their sets and assembled for sterilization and storage.

Forceps should be checked carefully to see that the tips are aligned correctly and that any ratchet grips are sound. Needle holders can be tested by lifting threads to test their grip. Scissors must be sharp, the tips easily cutting four thicknesses of gauze sponges.

Sterilization and disinfection

The recognition that pyogenic bacterial contamination is the cause of wound sepsis is of basic importance in surgery. *Asepsis* means the absence of any contamination of wounds, tissues or equipment. *Antisepsis* is the use of an agent to destroy or inhibit the growth of microorganisms in living tissues and may be achieved by the topical application of bactericidal or bacteriostatic agents to the tissues (anti-septics). Since spores are frequently unaffected by such treatment, the term disinfection is generally assumed to mean the destruction of vegetative forms. *Sterilization* on the other hand means the complete destruction of all types of microorganisms. This definition and the understanding of the fundamentals of sterilization are important in establishing and recognizing that many of the standard procedures that are used in practice in the field, e.g. the kettle boiling system, are not methods of sterilization and that in reality most of the procedures we carry out are *not* performed *aseptically*.

Factors that affect the sterilization process:

1 All material and instruments that need to be sterilized must be cleansed before sterilization.

2 Protein, bacteria and soap protect them from heat. Proteins may also inhibit many chemical disinfectants.

3 Old colonies are more resistant than young colonies and spores are much more resistant than vegetative forms.

In the practical sense, the two most important physical factors that influence the sterilization procedure are the concentration and temperature of chemical agents and the time of their application.

Dry heat

This may be achieved by direct flaming or in a hot air oven. The hot air oven may be used to sterilize instruments that would be damaged by moist heat. These processes may be effective, but they do, in fact, have disadvantages in that they are relatively slow.

Moist heat

This is by far the most commonly used system of sterilization in surgical practice. The most widely used agent is steam under pressure and it is used for all surgical instruments, dressings and appliances (autoclave). The manufacturer's instruction manual should be consulted for the recommended procedures. Built into the holding times will be a 25% safety factor, so that 15 min at 121°C with a steam pressure of 1.06 kg/cm^2(30 lb/in^2), 10 min at 126°C 1.4 kg/cm^2 (20 lb/in^2), or 3 min at 134°C and 2.1 kg/cm^2 (30 lb/in^2) are the criteria used. The sterilization cycle in a gravity displacement sterilizer is as follows. Firstly, there is steam entry and air removal. During this time air and condensate flow out through the chamber drain and penetration of steam into the load (if fabrics are being sterilized) commences. Secondly, the sterilization is then timed from when the chamber drain thermometer has reached the correct temperature. Thirdly, a partial vacuum is applied to remove moisture from the load and finally sterile air is admitted through a filter to break the vacuum.

For any load where penetration of steam is easy, such as unwrapped bottles, instruments or bottled fluids, gravity displacement sterilizers are effective and because of their relative simplicity are easy to maintain in good working order. It has been shown though that for instruments, although steam gains access to most surfaces with ease, box joints cannot be penetrated so easily. In order to ensure sterility of such sites sterilization at 149°C (50 lb/in^2) is recommended. As long as this temperature is reached in not less than 1 min, no holding time at 149°C is necessary, thus enabling the sterilizing cycle to be very short and in the order of 3–4 min.

For loads such as fabrics or rubber gloves where penetration is slow and can easily be prevented by incorrect packing, gravity displacement sterilizers are being superceded by a more efficient sterilizer that incorporates a prevacuum to remove air from the load. As such they are termed high prevacuum sterilizers. Such devices are used in hospitals but are unlikely to have use in general veterinary practice at the present time.

Gas sterilization

Bacteria are destroyed by aklylation. Formaldehyde was used but is now mostly replaced by ethylene oxide. Penetration of fabrics can be enhanced by a vacuum cycle. Ethylene oxide is toxic and damages rubber tubing. It is widely used to sterilize heat-sensitive equipment, e.g. endoscopes.

Chemical disinfection

This is employed where heat sterilization is impracticable. The action and efficacy is affected by:

1 The number and conditions of microorganisms present.

2 The nature of the surface to be disinfected.

3 The concentration and temperature of the agent that is being used.

4 The pH of the suspending medium, e.g. cationics are more active in alkaline solutions and anionics in acidic solution.

Many different agents are used:

Halogens—iodine and chlorine are the most commonly used halogens. A 1% solution of iodine kills all vegetative forms in 20 s. Iodine as a tincture is liable to be irritant to the skin, but iodophors (iodine plus non-ionic detergent) are non-staining and non-irritant.

Coal tars—phenols and cresols are often used as 'official' disinfectants but have little place in surgery.

Alcohols—ethyl alcohol is effective only as the 70% solution and is used alone or as the vehicle for iodine or iodophor.

Hexachlorophane—a phenol derivative; it is insoluble in water and is activated by soap. Used in a detergent (Phisohex) or as a pure sodium soap (Zalpon or Steridermis), it is applied to the clean dry hands and rubbed into the skin. Subsequent wetting gives a lather and causes hexachlorophane to be deposited into the skin pores thus giving a prolonged effect.

Glutaraldehyde—is used as 2% solution (Cide). It is rapid, effective and ideal for endoscopic equipment and endotracheal tubes.

Detergents

Quarternary ammonium, cationic, benzalkonium (Roccal,

Zephiran) centrimide (Cetavlon) and chlorhexidine (Hibitane) are used for skin and wound disinfection and for instrument storage.

Packaging prior to sterilization and storage is most important. Forceps should be secured in bundles and points and blades should be covered to prevent accidental penetration of the package. Packages must be labelled, dated and marked with sterilized safety tape or monitors (Fig. 9). Instruments, drapes and gloves for autoclaving may be packaged in nylon bags, or paper (Kraft) bags. Ethylene oxide will not penetrate either nylon or paper and material should be packed in polyethylene bags and sealed.

Instrument packs (Figs 1–6)

Basic set (spay set) (Fig. 1)

1 Stainless steel tray
1 Rat-tooth thumb forceps
1 Russian thumb forceps
1 Brown–Adson thumb forceps
2 Bard–Parker scalpel handle No. 3
3 Carmalt forceps
3 Rochester–Péan forceps
8 Backhaus towel clamps
4 Allis tissue forceps
3 Straight and 3 curved Halsted Mosquito artery forceps
Spay hook
1 Straight and 1 curved 6-inch Mayo scissors
1 8-inch curved Metzenbaum scissors
1 Mayo–Hegar needle holder

Wound or suture pack

1 Rat-tooth tissue forceps
1 Bard–Parker No. 3 scalpel handle
3 Curved Mosquito artery forceps (Halsted)
3 Straight Mosquito artery forceps (Halsted)
1 Curved Mayo scissors
4 Allis tissue forceps
4 Backhaus towel clamps

Thoracotomy set (Fig. 2)

Basic surgery set
Finochietto rib retractor
Malleable retractors
Mixter right angle artery forceps
Satinsky caval clamp/Knapp–Beck bronchus clamp
8-inch Metzenbaum scissors
10-inch needle holders

Orthopaedic set (Fig. 3)

Basic set	Osteotome
Jacob's chuck	Periosteal elevator
Pin drill	Bone rasp
Bone-holding forceps	ASIF basic set (Fig. 4)
Rongeurs	ASIF screw set (Fig. 5)
Kirschner wires	ASIF plating set (Fig. 6)
Wire twister	Power tools
Steinmann pins	

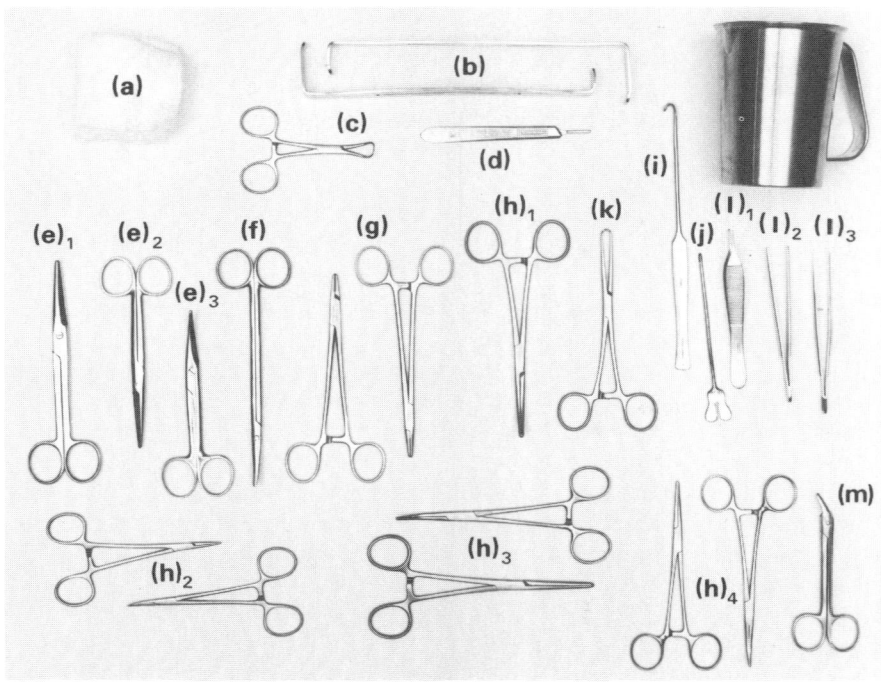

Fig. 1. Basic set. (a) Sponges; (b) Senn retractors; (c) Backhaus towel forceps; (d) Bard–Parker scalpel handle; (e)₁ straight Mayo scissors (blunt points); (e)₂ suture scissors (sharp, blunt points); (e)₃ curved Mayo scissors (blunt points); (f) Metzenbaum scissors; (g) Mayo–Hegar needle holders; (h)₁ Kelly artery forceps; (h)₂ straight and curved Mosquito artery forceps; (h)₃ Kocher artery forceps; (i) spay hook; (j) grooved director; (k) Allis tissue forceps; (l)₁ Brown–Adson thumb forceps; (l)₂ rat-tooth thumb forceps; (l)₃ Russian thumb forceps; (m) wire cutters.

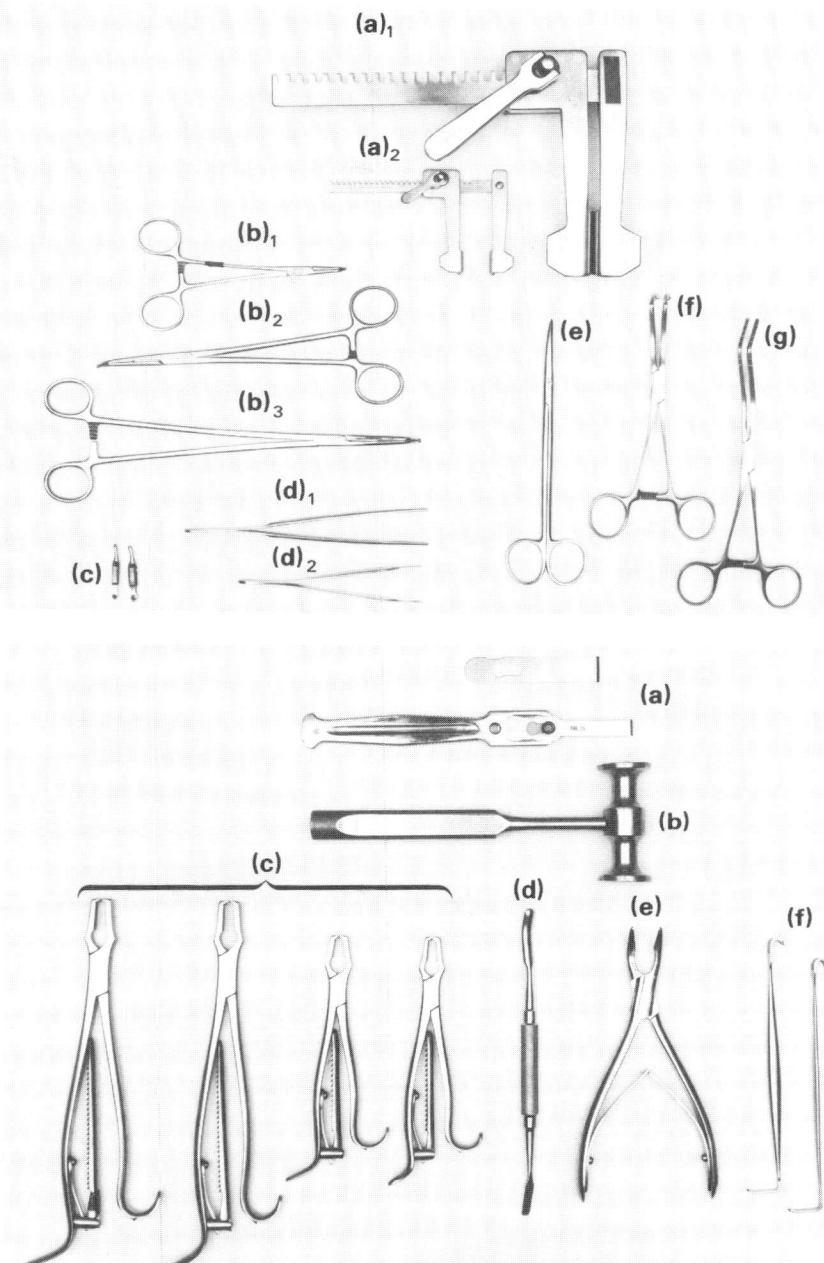

Fig. 2. Thoracotomy set. (a)$_1$Standard Finochietto rib retractor; (a)$_2$paediatric Finochietto rib retractor; (b)$_1$ Mixter right angle forceps, paediatric 14 cm; (b)$_2$ Mixter right angle forceps, standard 23 cm; (b)$_3$ Mixter right angle forceps, standard 28 cm; (c) Dieffenbach bulldog clips; (d)$_1$ Brown–Adson thumb forceps; (d)$_2$ Ewald thumb forceps; (e) Nelson scissors; (f) Satinsky caval clamp; (g) Kapp–Beck–Thompson bronchus clamp.

Fig. 3. Orthopaedic set. (a) Osteotome; (b) Richards bone hammer; (c) Lane bone holding forceps; (d) bone file; (e) Lempert rongeur; (f) Senn retractor—blade and hook ended.

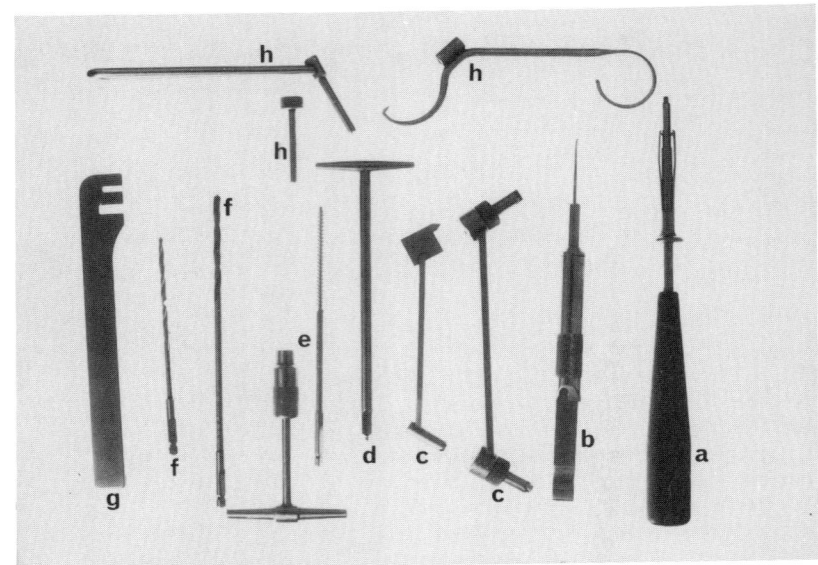

Fig. 4. ASIF instruments (3.5 mm system);
(a) Screwdriver; (b) depth gauge; (c) drill guides;
(d) countersink; (e) tap handle and tap; (f) drills;
(g) plate bending iron; (h) drill guides.

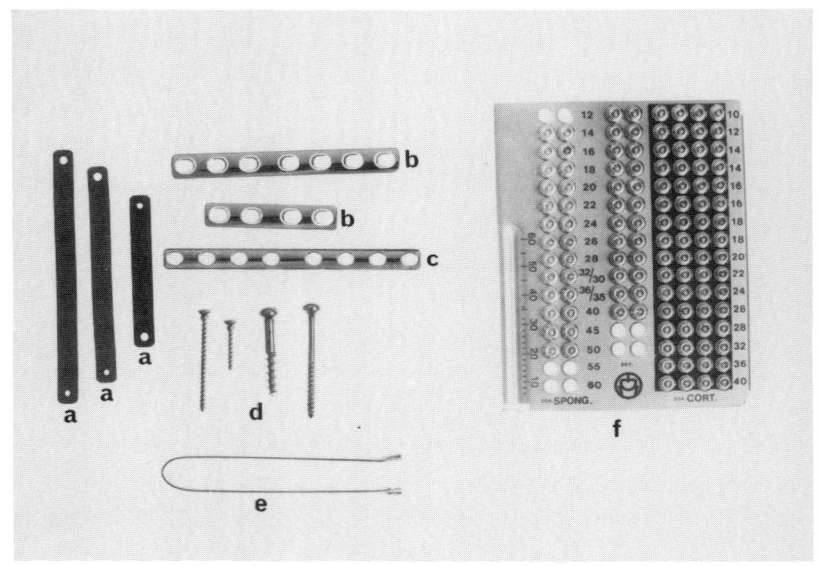

Fig. 5. ASIF screws and plates. (a) Plate
templates; (b) dynamic compression plates;
(c) semitubular plate; (d) cortical and cancellous
screws; (e) screw forceps; (f) screw rack.

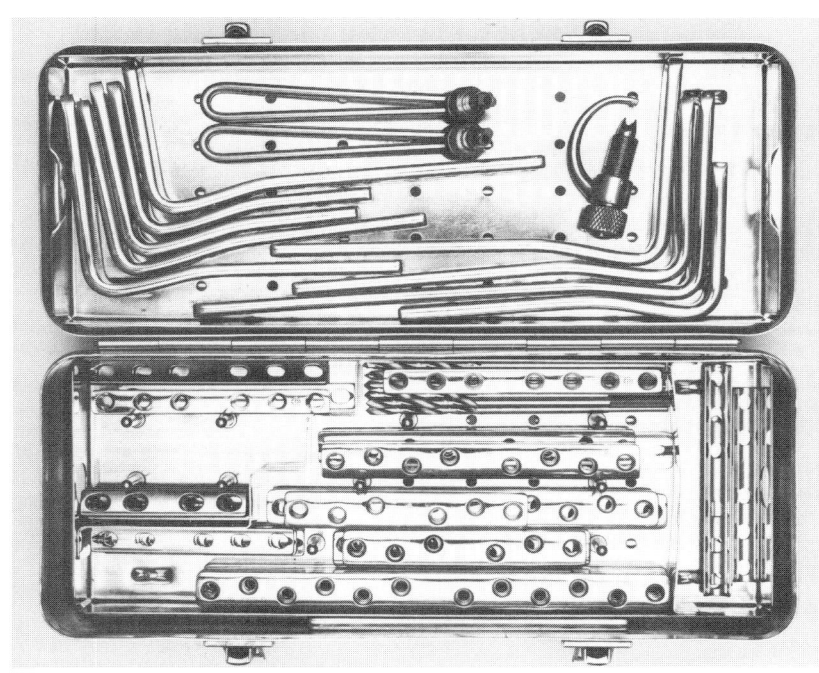

Fig. 6. ASIF plating set.

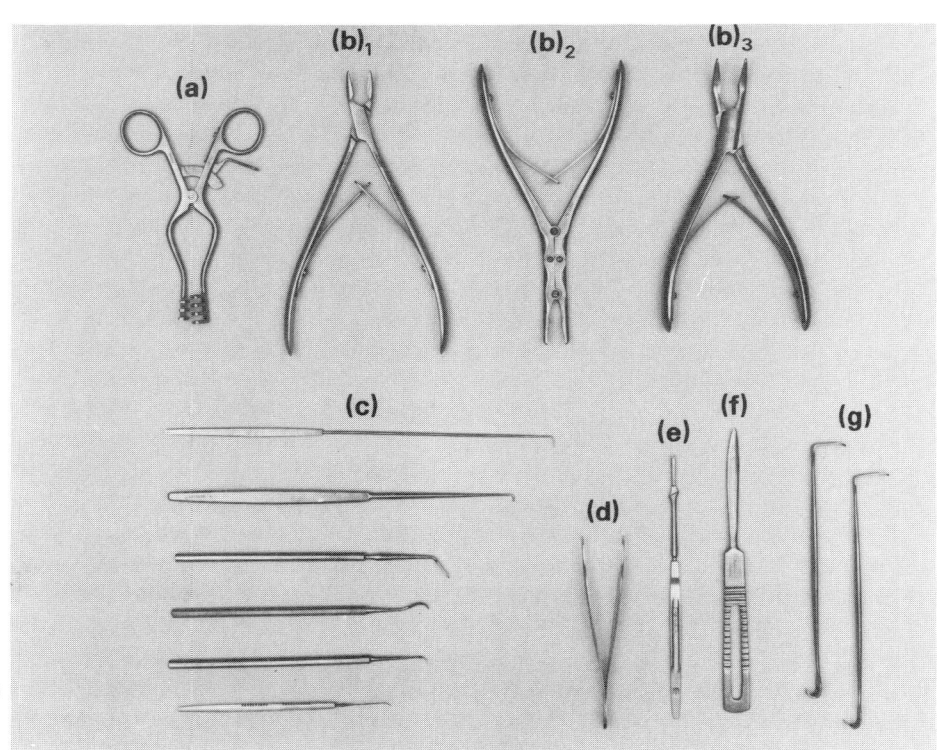

Fig. 7. (a) Weitlaner mastoid retractor; (b)$_1$ Lempert rongeur; (b)$_2$ Beyer rongeur; (b)$_3$ Lempert rongeur; (c) probes, picks and currettes (Gage); (d) Ewald thumb forceps; (e) Bard–Parker scalpel handle No. 7; (f) Bard–Parker periosteal elevator; (g) Senn retractor.

Laminectomy set (Fig. 7)

Basic set
Gelpi retractor (not illustrated)
Periosteal elevator
Weitlaner retractor
Lempert rongeur
Beyer rongeur
Hall power drill (not illustrated)

Fenestration hooks (Gage)
Currettes (Gage)

Basic ophthalmic set (Fig. 8)

Barraquer eye speculum
5-inch scissors
Pooley's conjunctival scissors
Castroviejo corneal scissors

Scalpel plus No. 12 blade
St Martin's forceps
Small rat-tooth forceps
Barraquer corneal forceps
Castroviejo needle holder
Halsted mosquito haemostats
Snellen's vectis

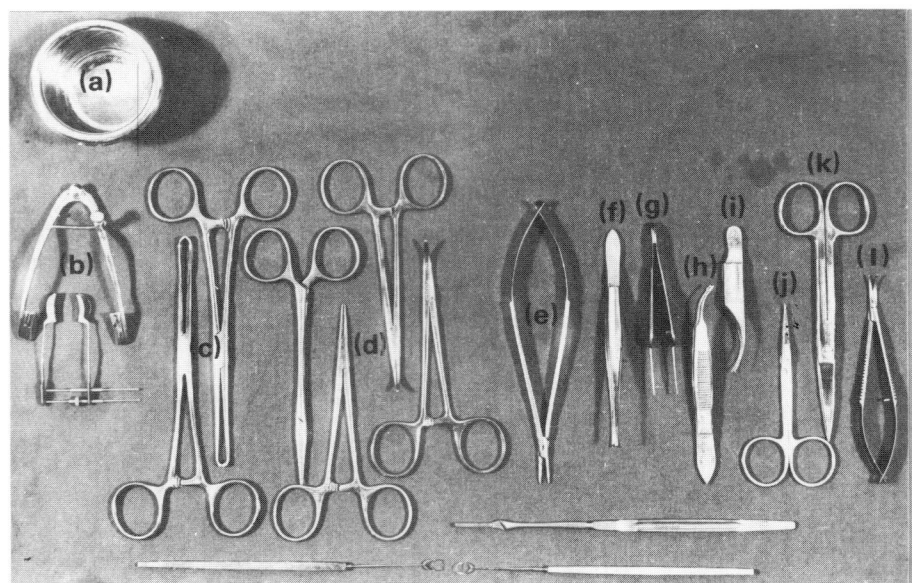

Fig. 8. Ophthalmic set. (a) Gallipot; (b) eyelid retractors; (c) Allis tissue forceps; (d) mosquito forceps—straight and curved; (e) Castroviejo needle holders; (f) rat-toothed dressing forceps; (g) St Martin's forceps; (h) Arruga's capsule forceps; (i) Barraquer forceps; (j) Pooley conjunctival scissors; (k) 4-inch scissors; (l) Castroviejo corneal scissors.

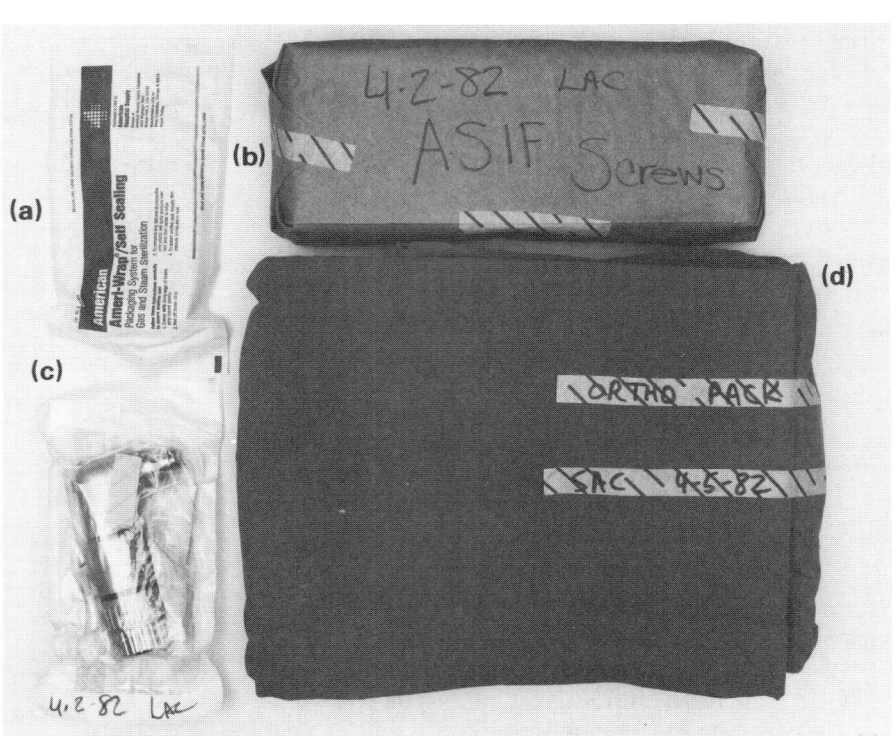

Fig. 9. Autoclaved surgical packs. (a) Paper; (b) paper; (c) nylon; (d) cloth wrapped steel tray. Note identification, date and heat sensitive marker tape.

Suture materials

It should remembered that all suture materials are foreign material, and as such, the body and tissues will react to them. To minimize tissue trauma and inflammation, the suture material used should be of the finest quality and of the finest calibre. Sutures should be placed with respect to tissue integrity. The use of sutures incorporating large bites of tissue, i.e. forming strangulation, must be prohibited. Suture material may be classified according to a number of properties; whether they are absorbable or non-absorbable, whether they are monofilament or multifilament or whether they are of a natural or synthetic product. It is convenient to use the absorbable/non-absorbable classification.

The ideal suture material should be strong, cheap, inert, easy to work with, giving good knot security. It should be easily sterilized and have a good shelf life. Obviously the ideal suture material does not exist, but major advances have been made in recent years to improve both the quality and range available.

Absorbable sutures

As originally defined, absorbable sutures were sterile strands prepared from mammalian collagen, catgut being the most widely used. However, the introduction of synthetic absorbable materials, Dexon (1960) (Davis & Geck) and Vicryl (1975) (Ethicon) has amended that definition.

Catgut is a twisted strand of collagen derived from the submucosa of ovine or the serosa of bovine small intestine. It is treated with chromium salts to delay phagocytosis within the tissues. Within 7 days embedded chromic catgut has lost 60% of its holding strength. Complete absorption by phagocytosis may, however, take several weeks or even months. Other natural collagen materials that can be used include tendon and fascia.

The first synthetic absorbable suture to be developed was PGA (polyglycolic acid—Dexon) which is a polymer of glycolic acid. Fine fibres of the material are braided into strands of varying thickness. This process produces a suture material that is very strong, easy to handle, fully absorbed and entirely excreted. The sutures are inert, non-antigenic and non-pyrogenic. PGA sutures are absorbed by hydrolysis and absorption is minimal until 14 days after implantation so that at 7 days there is 80% strength retention. It is entirely removed by 100–120 days. Polyglactin 910 (Vicryl) is a copolymer of glycolide and lactide. Its physical properties in handling and absorption are similar to the PGA. However, it is less hydrophylic because of the presence of methyl groups projecting from the polymer chain and dilaclide units.

Non-absorbable sutures

Natural fibres such as silk, linen and cotton have good tensile strength but are abrasive. They all have capillary attraction and should not be used in skin. Wire may be stainless steel, silver or tantalium, and is available in monofilament and braided forms. Nylons (polyamides) may be monofilament or multifilament and are non-capillary in the monofilament form. Its 50% strength life exceeds 6 months. Monofilament nylon has wide use in veterinary surgery, despite its rather brittle nature, and is an excellent skin and fascia suture. The newer synthetics are made of polyolefins (Dermalene, Davis & Geck) and polyesters (Dacron, Ticron, Davis & Geck; Tevdek, Ethibond, Ethicon). The teflon-coated products give poor knot security and at least four throws are recommended on all knots.

In some situations, non-absorbable sutures may be excreted. In the crushing bowel suture fine nylon is used and the suture may be shed into the bowel. Similarly silk may extrude from in the oral cavity and ultra-fine non-absorbable sutures may fragment and be phagocytosed.

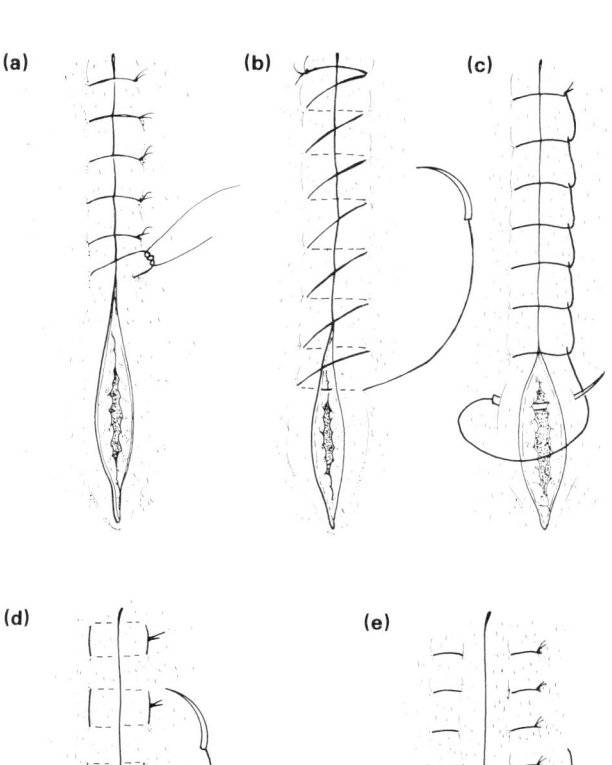

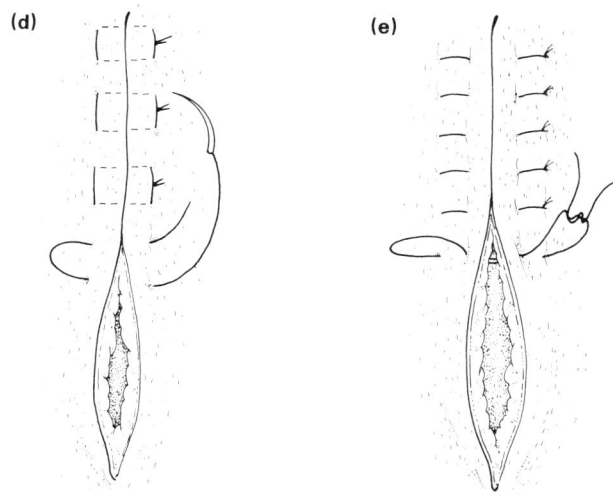

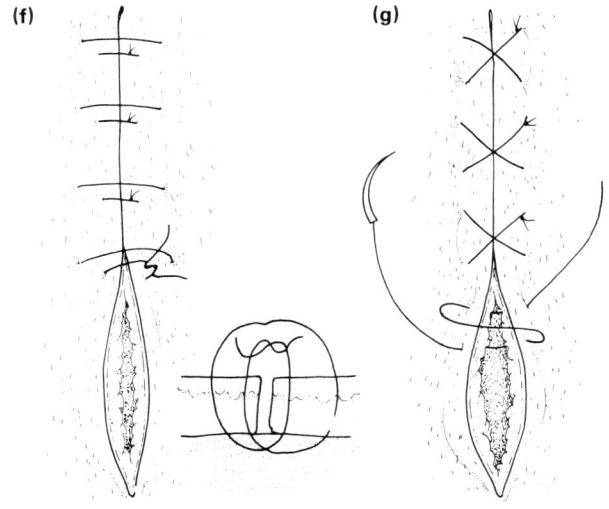

Fig. 10. Suture patterns: skin. (a) Simple interrupted; (b) simple continuous; (c) continuous lock; (d) horizontal mattress—interrupted; (e) vertical mattress; (f) near-far-near; (g) cruciate.

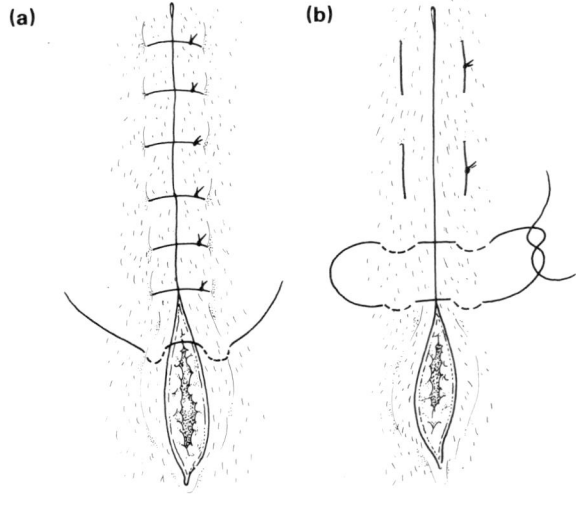

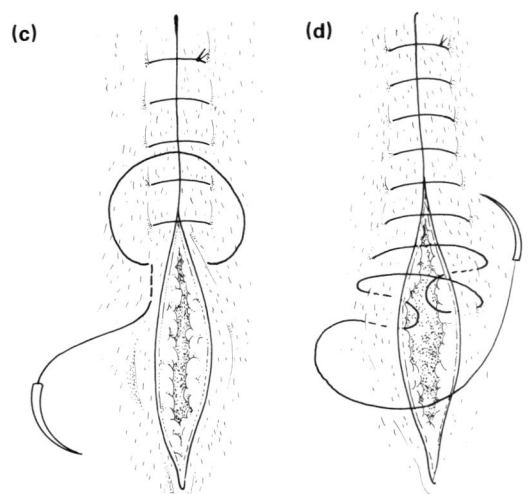

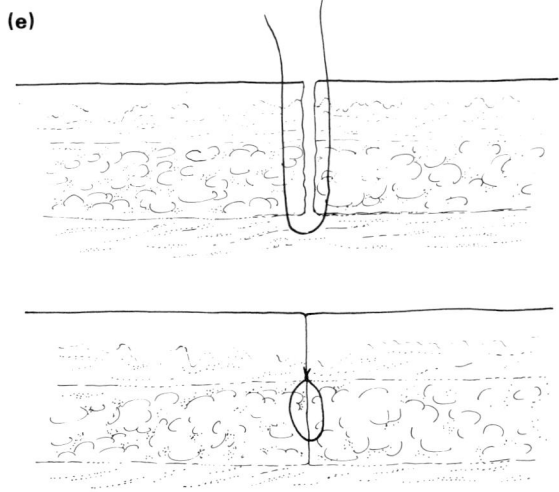

Suggested suture sizes and types for use in the dog (After Bellenger, 1982)

Tissue	Suture size (metric)	Suture type
Skin	1.0–0.7	Monofilament polypropylene and nylon; coated braided sutures of polyester or nylon
Fascia	3.5–2.0	Nylon; polypropylene; polyester or stainless steel
Gastrointestinal	2.0–1.5	Chromic gut; nylon; polypropylene
Urinary tract	2.0–1.5	Chromic gut; SA
Uterus	2.0–1.5	Chromic gut; SA
Tendon	3.5–2.0	Nylon; carbon fibre; stainless steel
Ligatures	3.0–2.0	Chromic gut; SA
Vascular structures	1.0–0.7	Polypropylene; nylon; silk; coated polyester

SA = Synthetic absorbable.

Suture patterns

Skin sutures

A variety of patterns are available for use in small animal surgery. In each case, the finest suture material should be used to appose and not compress the tissue—suture loose *knot* tight (Fig. 10a–10g).

Visceral sutures

The basic pattern is inversion to appose serosal surfaces; as shown by Halsted and others it is the serosal surface that affords a seal. In most instances a single row is all that is needed.

Modifications include the crushing intestinal anastomosis suture and the Gambee (Fig. 11a–11g).

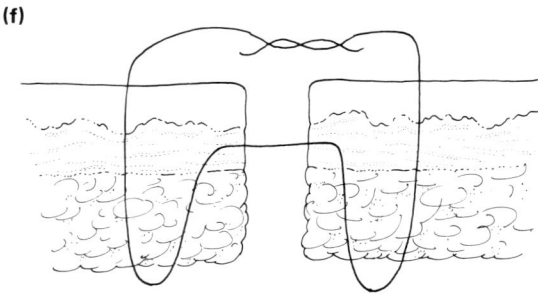

Fig. 11. Suture patterns: visceral sutures.
(a) Lembert; (b) Halsted; (c) Cushing;
(d) Connell; (e) Crushing; (f) Gambee.

Part B
Anaesthesia and Fluid Therapy

NICHOLAS H. DODMAN

Introduction

The purpose of this chapter is to review current methods of chemical restraint and anaesthesia in dogs and to relate them to the circumstances in which they may be most usefully employed. It includes notes on preoperative and intraoperative techniques and supportive measures. Anaesthetic apparatus, the treatment of emergencies occurring under anaesthesia and fluid therapy will also be discussed.

Anaesthesia

Preoperative evaluation of the patient

An estimate of the degree of risk involved in the anaesthesia of a particular patient can be made on the basis of history and clinical examination. A brief preoperative examination should be carried out with the salient points from the history in mind. A history suggestive of systemic disease or abnormal findings in the preoperative examination will necessitate a more detailed investigation before anaesthesia is undertaken.

Preoperative preparation of the patient

Routine preparation involves withholding food for 12 h and water for about 2 h before the induction of anaesthesia. When systemic disease or trauma causes a derangement in the normal physiology of the patient, appropriate preoperative preparation will decrease the anaesthetic risk and increase the likelihood of a speedy and uneventful recovery.

Cardiac disease

When cardiac disease is accompanied by exercise intolerance, the animal must be considered as a poor anaesthetic risk. In cases of chronic congestive cardiac failure, cage rest and diuretics can bring about a dramatic improvement. Digoxin may be indicated.

Pulmonary disease

There are two categories of pulmonary disease—obstructive and restrictive.

Obstructive pulmonary disease (e.g. bronchitis) is best treated by cage rest, broad-spectrum antibiotic therapy and bronchodilators. Improvement may take several days, but is worth waiting for if surgery can be delayed. Restrictive pulmonary disease is not always as amenable to therapy. Where the restriction results from an accumulation of fluid or air within the intrapleural space, thoracocentesis can bring about prompt relief of respiratory embarrassment and should be performed prior to anaesthesia.

Renal disease

The most common form of renal disease is chronic interstitial nephritis. The key to the successful management of these patients is the maintenance of an adequate fluid balance. Such patients have an inability to produce concentrated urine and will rapidly become uraemic if water intake is curtailed. They must be allowed free access to water until the time of premedication to meet their increased fluid requirements. An intravenous drip of an isotonic eletrolyte solution is advisable during surgery and should be continued until normal drinking starts again. Failure to observe these simple precautions can result in a uraemic crisis which usually takes the form of progressive post-operative malaise which may result in death a few days after surgery.

Hepatic disease

Very little can be done to improve the condition of patients with advanced hepatic disease. If the condition is acute and is likely to resolve with treatment then surgery should be delayed. Emergency surgery in this category of patient is extremely hazardous.

Pancreatic disease

Dogs with a history of exercise intolerance or collapsing should have blood glucose estimations performed prior to surgery. Should an abnormally low blood glucose level be detected, the preoperative preparation must include an intravenous infusion of 5–10% glucose, and monitoring of the blood glucose level both before and after surgery is necessary.

Stabilized diabetics should have their blood glucose level carefully monitored during anaesthesia. An intravenous drip of 10% glucose should be set up before anaesthesia and soluble insulin should be on hand. The blood glucose level is kept as near normal as possible by titrating insulin or glucose as necessary. If anaesthesia can be scheduled for early in the day, the patient can be given its usual dose of insulin as soon as it has recovered, and then allowed to eat.

Trauma cases

The preoperative therapy depends on the extent of the trauma. Less severe cases such as simple long bone fractures often require no specific treatment, but in such cases it is better to delay surgery for a few days to allow some resolution of the body fluid derangements which accompany bruising and haematoma formation. However, patients with multiple severe injuries will require extensive preanaesthetic therapy directed principally at the restoration and maintenance of normal cardiopulmonary function and the control of pain. Once again, it is better to delay surgery for a few days if possible to permit cardio-vascular stabilization and some resolution of conditions such as pulmonary contusion and mild pneumothorax.

Preanaesthetic medication

Premedication is an important part of any anaesthetic regime. Its purpose is to make the whole anaesthetic process safer and more pleasant for the patient. The types of drugs used include sedatives, narcotic analgesics and parasympatholytics.

Sedatives

These (a) facilitate induction and maintenance of anaesthesia, (b) reduce anaesthetic requirements, and (c) help to make recovery smoother.

1 *Acepromazine.* This is widely used:

Dose rate 0.05–0.1 mg/kg body weight i.m. or i.v.

Mild sedation with maximum effect lasting for about 2 h.

Should be avoided or at least used with caution in hypovolaemic patients.

In patients with marked sinus arrhythmia at rest, acepromazine can cause syncopy associated with profound bradycardia (atropine given at the same time as acepromazine will prevent such a crisis).

Lowers the seizure threshold in epileptics (it is best to avoid acepromazine in dogs which have a history of fits).

The adrenolytic and hypothermic activity of acepromazine reduces the body temperature during anaesthesia.

Certain breeds of dogs (e.g. Boxer, Irish Setter) seem to be unduly susceptible to the central sedative action of acepromazine. This in itself is not a major problem but it should be born in mind that a reduced dose is often adequate.

2 *Xylazine.* This offers some advantages over acepromazine:

More profound sedation.

More reliable effect.

One problem associated with its use is that it causes vomition in a significant proportion of patients. Proper fasting, atropine premedication and a low dose rate of xylazine (0.5 mg/kg i.m.) will considerably reduce the problem. Because of its emetic properties, xylazine is contraindicated in patients with intestinal obstruction.

Produces bradycardia and a transient rise in blood pressure. The bradycardia can be prevented by pretreatment with atropine.

Narcotic analgesics

Used as premedicants either (a) to supplement intra-operative analgesia when balanced anaesthetic techniques are used, or (b) for their analgesia effect during recovery when moderate to severe pain is anticipated following surgery.

Drugs commonly used for this purpose are morphine, pethidine and pentazocine.

1 *Morphine.* The following can be said:

Probably still the drug of choice because of its sustained action (up to 4 h).

The dose rate is 0.5 mg/kg body weight i.m.

2 *Pethidine.* The following can be said:

Uncommon usage in the dog.

The dose rate is up to 2 mg/kg body weight i.m.

3 *Pentazocine.* The following can be said:

Short duration in the dog.

The dose rate is 2 mg/kg body weight i.m.

Neuroleptanalgesic combinations

Combinations such as etorphine/methotrimeprazine (Small Animal Immobilon) and fentanyl/fluanisone (Hypnorm) can be used to premedicate fractious dogs. A lower dose rate is utilized than when they are used as sole agents for minor procedures. The dose rate of any intravenous induction agent used subsequently is reduced in proportion to the level of central nervous depression produced.

Parasympatholytics

1 *Atropine.* The most widely employed parasympatholytic agent in small animal anaesthetic practice:

Prevents or alleviates bradycardia of parasympathetic origin.

Reduces salivation.

Prevents the unwanted muscarinic effects of neostigmine when the latter is used to reverse competitive muscle relaxants.

The dose rate is 0.04 mg/kg body weight i.m., i.v. or s.c.

Some veterinary surgeons give atropine routinely prior to anaesthesia, but others prefer to reserve it for situations in which it is specifically indicated. The latter would seem to be a more reasonable approach, because there is some evidence that cardiac dysrhythmias of sympathetic origin are more likely when resting vagal tone has been abolished. The vagolytic effect is specifically required when surgery is likely to cause enhanced vagal activity (e.g. ocular surgery). Excessive salivation is rarely a problem during anaesthesia unless ether is used.

Induction of anaesthesia

Barbiturates

1 *Thiopentone.* With this anaesthetic:

The dose rate in healthy unpremedicated dogs is around 20 mg/kg body weight i.v.

Premedication with acepromazine reduces the induction dose to approximately 10 mg/kg body weight. The dose rate is even lower if xylazine has been used as the premedicant.

Cardiovascular disease, hepatic disease, renal disease, hypovolaemia, hypothyroidism, and old age all influence the dose/response relationship of thiopentone. In such instances it is best to give a small test dose and observe the effect.

Except for short procedures, thiopentone should not be used to maintain anaesthesia because it is cumulative. If more than two or three incremental doses have been used to maintain anaesthesia an undesirably prolonged recovery can result.

Certain breeds (Greyhounds, Salukis, Afghans) and young or emaciated animals can have a prolonged recovery from a single dose of thiopentone because of their relative lack of body fat.

Thiopentone is an irritant and perivascular injection can cause a serious slough. Such sloughs are less likely if a 2½% solution is used. Following perivascular injection the area should be infiltrated with saline or a local anaesthetic solution to reduce the risk of a slough.

2 *Methohexitone.* The following can be said:

A N-methyl barbiturate.

About twice as potent as thiopentone (the dose rate used in any situation is approximately half that of intravenous thiopentone).

Rapidly metabolized by the liver and so has an ultra-short duration of action.

Unconsciousness lasts for 5–8 min following a full anaesthetic dose.

Because of rapid metabolism it is not cumulative, and 'topping up' is quite acceptable as a method of prolonging anaesthesia.

Lacks significant tissue irritancy, and skin sloughs are unlikely following perivascular injection.

Will cause more respiratory depression than thiopentone.

Can cause tremors and excitement at induction and during recovery.

Excitement can be minimized by sedative premedication.

3 *Pentobarbitone.* There is no compelling reason why this drug should still be used. It has the advantage of producing medium duration (30 min) anaesthesia following a single intravenous injection of 30 mg/kg, but there is a prolonged recovery period.

Inhalational agents

There are some circumstances in which induction using inhalational agents may be preferable to the use of barbiturates.

A face-mask attached to an anaesthetic circuit is used. The safest and least disturbing method is to allow the animal to breathe pure oxygen first, then to increase the concentration of the inhalational agent gradually until a level sufficient to induce anaesthesia is attained. High flows are desirable because they cause rapid denitrogenation of the patient and allow more precise control of the inspired concentration. At induction the concentration of anaesthetic in the lungs is always lower than that indicated on the vaporizer but high fresh gas flows cause the alveolar concentration to approach that set on the vaporizer more rapidly. Agents used include ether, halothane, methoxy-flurane, enflurane, isoflurane, nitrous oxide, and cyclopropane.

Any inhalation agent can be used to induce anaesthesia. Halothane is probably the best that is currently available, and 3–4% halothane vapour in oxygen will induce anaesthesia in about 5 min or less. Isoflurane shows great promise for the future, there being even faster induction and recovery.

Maintenance of anaesthesia

Following induction it is usual to intubate the animal and maintain anaesthesia using an inhalational agent.

Spontaneous breathing techniques are satisfactory for the majority of anaesthetics, and the essence of such techniques is to maintain anaesthesia at the minimum level which is compatible with the surgery being performed. Balanced anaesthesia is safer for poor risk patients. Here, narcosis is produced using a low concentration of an inhalational agent, and muscle relaxation, together with the suppression of reflex movement are ensured by the use of a specific muscle relaxant drug. Intermittent positive pressure ventilation (IPPV) necessarily becomes an integral part of balanced anaesthesia because the muscles of respiration are paralysed.

Volatile liquids

1 *Diethyl ether.* The following can be said:

Safe, but has the disadvantage of being inflammable and explosive.

Has a pungent odour and is irritating to respiratory passages.

Respiration is stimulated in light planes of anaesthesia.

The cardiovascular system is relatively stable during anaesthesia.

Ether does not sensitize the heart to the effects of catecholamines.

Muscle relaxation is good during ether anaesthesia.

The effects of non-depolarizing muscle relaxants are potentiated.

The concentration of ether required to maintain anaesthesia is between 2–5%.

2 *Halothane.* This volatile liquid has the following properties:

Potent.

Non-irritant.

The respiratory system is depressed at all levels of halothane anaesthesia.

Arterial hypotension occurs during halothane anaesthesia (there is a direct relationship between depression of the blood pressure and the depth of the anaesthesia).

Has the undesirable property of sensitizing the heart to the effects of circulating catecholamines and this can result in cardiac arrhythmias.

3 *Methoxyflurane*. Can be described thus:

Its physical properties are such that the maximum vapour concentration which can be achieved under normal clinical conditions is about 3%.

High blood solubility makes induction and recovery relatively slow.

Postoperative analgesia is good.

It depresses respiration in proportion to the depth of anaesthesia.

The circulatory system remains fairly stable during anaesthesia.

The heart is minimally sensitized to catecholamines.

Maintenance concentration 0.3% (at equilibrium).

Potentially nephrotoxic as a result of biotransformation to free fluoride ion.

4 *Enflurane*. Has the following properties:

One of the new inhalational agents.

A potent non-inflammable inhalation anaesthetic which undergoes only minimal biotransformation.

Resembles methoxyflurane in its chemical structure but has properties which are more like halothane.

Induction of anaesthesia can be achieved rapidly using a 4–6% inspired concentration.

Anaesthesia can be maintained with a 2–3% concentration.

Muscle relaxation is good.

The heart is minimally sensitized to catecholamines.

The main disadvantage is the occurrence of muscular tonic–clonic twitching which can develop during anaesthesia. EEG changes indicate nervous irritability.

5 *Isoflurane*. Can be described in the following manner:

Has chemical and pharmacological properties comparable to those of halothane and enflurane.

Does not cause involuntary jerking or seizure activity characteristic of its isomer, enflurane.

Pungent odour.

Good muscle relaxation.

Less sensitization of the heart to catecholamines than occurs with halothane.

Induction and maintenance concentrations are similar to those of enflurane.

Gases

1 *Nitrous oxide*. The following can be said:

Colourless with a faint rather pleasant smell.

Not flammable or explosive.

Non-irritant.

Low toxicity.

Low potency (the MAC★ value in the dog is 188%).

Must be supplemented with another agent to maintain anaesthesia.

Rapid diffusion out of the blood can cause hypoxia in early recovery (give pure oxygen for 3 to 5 min after the nitrous oxide is turned off).

★The minimum alveolar concentration required to prevent response to a surgical stimulus in 50% of a group of test patients.

2 *Cyclopropane*. Can be described as follows:

Colourless with a garlic-like odour.

Inflammable and highly explosive when mixed with air or oxygen.

Cyclopropane has a low blood : gas solubility coefficient and is potent, so that induction of anaesthesia is rapid (the MAC value in the dog is 17.5%).

Recovery is rapid even after prolonged anaesthesia.

The heart is sensitized to the effects of circulating catecholamines and catecholamine production is also increased so that arrhythmias are common.

Muscle relaxants

Muscle relaxants are given intravenously to the unconscious patient to produce complete muscular relaxation, and abolish reflex movement. Since the intercostal muscles and the diaphragm are affected, IPPV is mandatory. The idea of using muscle relaxants during surgery is daunting to many practitioners but there is no good reason for this since, in essence, all that is required is an extra injection and intermittent squeezing of the reservoir bag. By using muscle relaxants, surgery can be performed at a much lighter level of anaesthesia than would otherwise be possible, but *one must ensure that the unconscious state prevails*. An animal which is under the influence of muscle relaxants and which is on the verge of consciousness will show the following signs:

Lacrimation
Salivation
Tachycardia
Increase in blood pressure.

There are two types of muscle relaxants; the non-depolarizing (competitive) and the depolarizing.

The only *depolarizing muscle relaxant* used clinically is *succinylcholine*. In the dog, a dose rate of 0.3 mg/kg will produce up to 20 min paralysis. Within 30 s of the injection of the drug transient fasciculations are seen. Complete relaxation follows within 10–15 s. Neuromuscular transmission is resumed when a sufficient quantity of the drug has been hydrolysed by plasma cholinesterase to allow the repolarization of the postsynaptic membrane. Depolarizing muscle relaxants cannot be reversed. Succinylcholine can be used as the muscle relaxant component of balanced anaesthesia, with supplementary doses being given at approximately 20 minute intervals to maintain relaxation. Supplementary doses should be ⅓ of the original dose.

Non-depolarizing relaxants last in excess of 30 min and can be effective for up to an hour, depending on the relaxant used and the dose given. *Pancuronium* is popular currently, and, at a dose rate of 0.08 mg/kg, will produce relaxation of sufficient duration for most surgical procedures. Like other non-depolarizing muscle relaxants, its action must be reversed at the end of a procedure by the administration of a small dose of neostigmine i.v. The neostigmine is titrated incrementally until spontaneous respiration is resumed. Before the neostigmine is administered, atropine should be given i.v. to counteract the unwanted muscarinic effects of the drug.

Anaesthetic machines and circuits

Anaesthetic machines

The basic components of any anaesthetic machine are gas cylinders, reducing valves, a flowmeter bank and one or more vaporizers.

Gas cylinders (size E)

1 Oxygen cylinders—colour-coded black with small white section at the valve end; compressed gas in cylinder; contents gauge indicates amount present.
2 Nitrous oxide cylinders—colour-coded blue; liquid in cylinder; contents of cylinder assessed by weighing.

All cylinders are pin-indexed so that they can only be attached to the correct yoke on the machine.

The reducing valves

They have the following functions:
To step down the pressure in the cylinder to a more manageable level.
To make frequent adjustments of the flowmeter unnecessary by causing it to be presented with a relatively constant pressure head.
To make fine adjustment of the flowmeter easier.

The flowmeters

Most modern flowmeters are rotameters. They have the following characteristics:
Each one is calibrated for a particular gas and is only accurate for that gas.
The flow is controlled by a needle valve at the base of the flowmeter.
The rotameter tube tapers, so that it is wider at the top than the bottom.
The higher the bobbin floats in the tube, the wider is the annular space around it and consequently the greater the flow.
Accuracy ±2%.
Affected by tilting and static electricity.

Vaporizers

A good vaporizer 'makes' an anaesthetic machine. Ideally it should be calibrated and should be accurate over a wide range of flow rates. It should not give an initial high concentration of vapour when first turned on and should not be affected by movement, back pressure or changes in temperature of the anaesthetic it contains. The Fluotec Mark III is such a vaporizer. It is a temperature- and flow-compensated vaporizer for halothane which is calibrated in percent halothane and is accurate over prolonged periods of use even during IPPV. Vaporizers of this type are available for use with methoxyflurane (Pentec, Cyprane Ltd) ether (Ethertec, Cyprane Ltd) and enflurane (Enfluratec, Cyprane Ltd). Ideally they should be serviced every year to maintain them in optimum condition.

Anaesthetic circuits

The circuits are either closed or semi-closed.

Closed circuits

The essential features are:
Fresh gas inlet.
Carbon dioxide absorber.
Reservoir bag.
Unidirectional values (for circle arrangement).

Oxygen is added to the circuit to meet the patient's metabolic requirements and carbon dioxide is absorbed by soda lime granules in the absorber. A small amount of anaesthetic has to be added to the circuit along with the fresh gas in order to maintain anaesthesia because there is continuous uptake of the agent from the lungs throughout the whole period of anaesthesia.

The two arrangements which can be used for closed circuit anaesthesia are the to-and-fro and the circle.
1 To-and-fro. Advantages: less resistance than circle; easily sterilized.
Disadvantages: apparatus dead space progressively increases throughout anaesthesia as soda lime is used up; inhalation of irritant dust; some of the respired gases may bypass the soda lime unless the cylinder is packed tight.
2 Circle. Advantages: apparatus dead space (from endotracheal type to Y-connector) remains constant; little risk of irritant dust inhalation.
Disadvantage: regular size of circle should not be used in animals less than 15 kg bodyweight because of resistance to gas flow and poor mixing of gases.

Semi-closed anaesthesia

There are two arrangements which can be used; with absorption, and without absorption:
1 With absorption. Both to-and-fro and circle circuits can be used as semi-closed circuits. To do this, a valve in the circuit is opened and the fresh gas flow rate is increased above that required for a closed circuit, so that there is a constant spill of gas from the valve. The concentration of anaesthetic in the circuit approaches (but never reaches) the vaporizer concentration if the vaporizer is outside the circuit. The increased fresh gas flow rate makes this system

more responsive, so that it is easier to control the depth of anaesthesia. This advantage is only achieved at the expense of increased wastage of anaesthetic and oxygen and increased theatre pollution (unless gases are scavenged).

2 *Without absorption.* The second type of semi-closed circuit relies on high fresh gas flow rates in order to wash away expired carbon dioxide and does not, therefore, require the presence of a soda lime absorber. These circuits have negligible apparatus dead space and low resistance to gas flow making them suitable for small dogs and cats.

Ayre's T-piece (Fig. 12). This particular system requires a fresh gas flow of twice the patient's minute respiratory volume (minute respiratory volume = kg body weight × 0.2 l). During expiration fresh gas and expired gas pass into a reservoir tube. During the expiratory pause fresh gas flushes this mixture of gases out of the reservoir tube. The volume of the reservoir tube must be at least equal to the tidal volume to prevent atmospheric air from being entrained. A useful modification of Ayre's T-piece is the addition of an open-ended reservoir bag at the distal end of the reservoir tube—this facilitates positive pressure ventilation and respiratory monitoring.

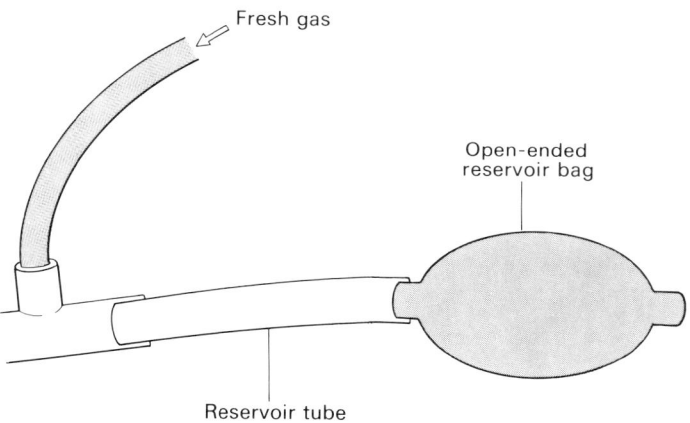

Fig. 12. Ayre's T-piece.

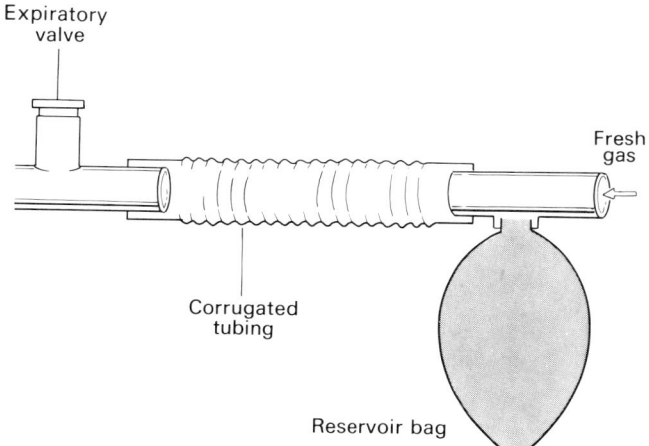

Fig. 13. Magill circuit.

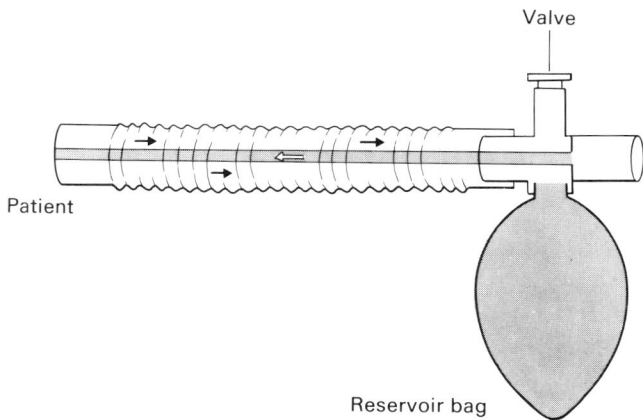

Fig. 14. Bain circuit (co-axial).

Magill circuit (Fig. 13). This circuit requires a fresh gas flow rate equal to the patient's minute respiratory volume. During expiration the expired gas passes back along the corrugated tube and some also escapes from the overflow valve. Expired gas never reaches the reservoir bag since the capacity of the corrugated tube is greater than the maximum expected tidal volume. During the expiratory pause fresh gas sweeps the expired gas out of the overflow valve.

Bain circuit (co-axial) (Fig. 14). This third type of semi-closed circuit without absorption has recently become available. It is best to think about this circuit as a T-piece folded back on iself. The fresh gas is delivered through the inner co-axial tube whilst the annular space around it acts as the reservoir tube. This circuit is particularly useful when head or neck surgery is being performed since only a single lightweight tube connects the animal to the anaesthetic machine, making surgical access easier.

Anaesthetic accidents and emergencies

Shock

Shock is circulatory failure. During surgery it can arise as a result of untreated blood loss. If the blood loss is less than 15% of the blood volume, and if the autonomic reflexes responsible for the relocation of the blood volume are not impaired by undue depth of anaesthesia, the cardiac output and systemic arterial blood pressure can be maintained for a while by reflex mechanisms. Even so it is good practice to replace losses as they occur, otherwise shock can become refractory to treatment.

Cardiac arrest

In most cases cardiac arrest is reversible and survival can be expected if prompt and efficient treatment is given. The most important factor in the treatment of the condition is the speed at which restorative measures are instituted.

The factors predisposing to cardiac arrest are:
Hypoventilation.
Hypovolaemia.
Hypothermia.
Increased parasympathetic tone.
Increased sympathetic tone.

Prophylactic measures

1 Ensure an adequate airway by means of a cuffed endotracheal tube.
2 Make sure that the inspired anaesthetic mixture contains at least 30% oxygen.
3 Replace blood loss occurring during the operation.
4 Use a heating pad for animals under 5 kg.
5 Premedicate with atropine when vagal stimulation is a possibility.
6 Preanaesthetic sedative drugs should be given to minimize excitement on induction.

Signs of cardiac arrest

1 Cessation of voluntary respiration.
2 Absence of peripheral pulse.
3 Dilation of pupil.
4 Absence of heart sounds on auscultation.
5 Cyanosis or pallor of mucous membranes.
6 No bleeding at operation site.

Management

1 Ventilation with O_2.
2 External cardiac compression.
3 Internal cardiac compression (if external compression is ineffective).
4 Bicarbonate—the pH drops to 7 within a minute or so. This should be corrected with 8.4% sodium bicarbonate solution—1–1.5 ml/kg/body weight i.v. as fast as possible. Thereafter, 0.1 ml/min/kg/body weight i.v.
   There are two types of cardiac arrest: asystole and ventricular fibrillation. The initial treatment for both is as described but ancillary therapy differs. Asystole may respond to intravenous or intracardiac adrenaline (1:10,000 dilution). Fibrillation is best treated by direct current electrical defibrillation.

Arrhythmias

Disturbances in cardiac rhythm can be encountered at any stage of anaesthesia. They are frequently innocuous and go unnoticed unless there is constant ECG monitoring. Those which are clinically significant are the extreme tachyarrhythmias and the extreme bradyarrhythmias. Arrhythmias associated with increased sympathetic activity are more likely in the presence of certain inhalational anaesthetics which 'sensitize the heart' to the effects of adrenaline. Hypoxia and hypercapnia cause stimulation of the sympathetic nervous system, so arrhythmias are common when respiration is depressed. Many can be converted simply by establishing adequate respiratory exchange. Bradyarrhythmias can occur in any animal, but are commonly encounted in dogs with an increased resting vagal tone. Treatment with atropine is normally effective.

Ventilatory failure

Any factor which depresses either the respiratory centre, nervous transmission to the muscles of respiration or the free movement of the thoracic wall (including the diaphragm) predisposes to ventilatory failure. In a patient breathing air this causes hypoxaemia and hypercapnia. However, if an oxygen-enriched amosphere is being breathed, as during inhalational anaesthesia, hypercapnia may present on its own. The treatment is to ventilate the lungs with oxygen while the cause of the ventilatory failure is corrected.

Laryngospasm

Laryngospasm is unusual in the dog. It is caused by mechanical or chemical stimulation of the larynx in light anaesthesia and, although normally self-limiting, can result in a potentially dangerous degree of hypoxia (with associated hypercapnia). Furthermore, pulmonary oedema can result from respiratory obstruction. Treatment of laryngospasm is by intubation and ventilation. This may require the prior administration of a muscle relaxant drug, and succinylcholine is used because of its relatively rapid action.

Vomition

Vomition occurs in light anaesthesia and it is usually heralded by jerking movements. The head and neck of the animal should be lowered to protect the airway. If aspiration occurs the airway must be cleared of debris and subsequent treatment with a broad spectrum antibiotic and corticosteroids should be instituted.

Perivascular injection of thiopentone

Accidental perivenous injection can cause massive tissue necrosis and sloughing. The treatment is to dilute the injected solution with a large volume of saline, or to inject an equal volume of a local anaesthetic solution into the site. The latter causes the thiopentone to precipitate.

Hypothermia

Hypothermia exists when the body core temperature falls below 35°C. It is one of the most common causes of a delayed return to consciousness in the small dog. For the body temperature to remain static, heat gain must equal heat loss. Hypothermia occurs during anaesthesia as a result of decreased heat production and increased heat loss. Decreased heat production is inevitable, but increased heat loss can be largely avoided.

Recommendations

1 Minimize conduction losses: heated water blanket, well-insulated table, avoid excessive wetting of skin.
2 Minimize evaporative losses: humidify operating theatre and inspired gas.
3 Warm all intravenous and lavage fluids.
4 Maintain high ambient temperature (22°C minimum).
5 Monitor body temperature in high risk patients.

Fluid therapy

Fluid and electrolyte balance in the normal animal

The normal dog produces approximately 20 ml urine/kg body weight per day. A similar volume of fluid is lost from the lungs and skin and in the faeces, making a total fluid output of 40 ml/kg body weight per day. The urinary loss of fluid is regulated by the release of antidiuretic hormone from the posterior pituitary gland which can significantly reduce urine output if circumstances demand. Loss of fluid from the lungs, however, continues even in the presence of severe dehydration and is termed insensible (or obligatory) water loss. The normal fluid output is balanced by an intake of 40 ml/kg body weight per day. Thirst determines the exact amount drunk and balance is achieved whereby:

Oral intake = urinary output + insensible water loss

Electrolyte homeostasis is under the control of the mineralocorticoid, aldosterone.

How deficiencies arise

Any condition which prevents an animal from drinking will lead to primary water depletion. This occurs relatively slowly in normal animals, but in animals which are polyuric as a result of chronic nephritis, diabetes mellitus or diabetes insipidus, input failure will rapidly result in a deficiency.

Excessive losses of fluid from the gastrointestinal tract involve the simultaneous loss of both water and electrolytes so that a complex deficit develops. Vomition is probably the most common cause of serious fluid imbalance. Animals with diarrhoea are usually able to compensate for fluid lost by increasing their oral intake of fluid but in time electrolyte disturbances notably hypokalaemia, can develop. The pyometra complex provides another example of simultaneous water and electrolyte loss since the uterine discharge is rich in ions.

Diagnosis of the disorder

The diagnosis of fluid and electrolyte depletion must be based on clinical history, physical examination and laboratory data.

History

Decreased intake of fluid or increased losses indicate the possibility of a fluid deficit. The type and likely extent of the deficit can be established by carefully questioning the owner regarding the animal's immediate antecedent clinical history. Important questions to ask are:
1 Is the animal drinking and managing to keep fluid down?
2 Is the animal passing urine?
3 Has the animal vomited or had diarrhoea? If so, how often and how much?
4 How long has the condition been present?

The answers to these questions are most important and can give the practitioner a good idea of the extent of the deficit.

Example: A 30 kg dog presents with a history of vomiting for 2 days. It is established by questioning the owner that the animal has also been adipsic and oliguric. The following losses have been incurred:

Insensible (20 ml/kg/day)	=	1200 ml
Urinary loss (estimated 10 ml/kg/day)	=	600 ml
Alimentary loss (estimated)	=	200 ml
Total loss	=	2000 ml

The example given above indicates the magnitude of fluid loss which can occur in a relatively short period of time.

Clinical examination

Loss of body fluid is manifested by clinical signs which indicate a volume deficit in each of the three body compartments. Intravascular fluid volume depletion gives rise to signs of shock, e.g. a fast, weak pulse, poor capillary refill time and cold extremities. Interstitial fluid depletion gives rise to a loss of tissue turgor with consequent looseness of the skin and sinking of the eyes. Intracellular volume depletion appears as an acute decrease in body weight.

Depending on the extent of the depletion these signs may be present to a greater or lesser degree. In advanced cases patients become dull and weak and may eventually become comatose.

Simple laboratory determinations

These tests may be diagnostic but, in general, are only confirmatory. The packed cell volume, plasma protein level and blood urea level are usually elevated in dehydration. Although these determinations are useful, the results must be interpreted with a degree of caution since anaemia, hypoproteinaemia and renal disease, respectively, can cause some confusion. Checking the urine specific gravity with a hydrometer or refractometer can also be of value. Levels are usually greater than 1.035 in dehydration.

Clinical examination and laboratory determinations should be repeated regularly throughout treatment to check that there is an improvement in the animal's condition.

Treatment

When fluid replacement therapy has been deemed necessary, the first step is to insert an indwelling catheter into a superficial vein. The cephalic or the jugular veins are most frequently used. To prevent clotting the catheter is primed with heparanized saline before its attachment to the drip unit.

The next step is to connect up the appropriate replacement solution to the catheter by means of an administration set. Although a standard blood administration set can be used for large dogs, it is probably better to practice to use an administration set incorporating a burette chamber so that accurate volume replacement can be performed (this is particularly important for small dogs).

The choice of solution to be used always seems to cause some confusion but this need not be so if the objectives of fluid therapy are understood. These objectives are:
1 To provide daily maintenance needs.
2 To repair deficits developed prior to treatment.
3 To replace any concurrent abnormal losses.

If it is remembered that maintenance needs are required to balance insensible water loss and urinary water loss, and that only small amounts of electrolytes are lost by these routes, then it will become apparent that only a dilute electrolyte solution is required for this purpose. A fifth normal saline solution (0.18%) is adequate for short-term maintenance therapy.

In replacing existing deficits it is first necessary to ascertain what losses have been incurred and then to consider each loss individually. If only water has been lost in, for example, a case of heat stroke, then only water is needed for replacement. Five per cent dextrose solution is usually used for this purpose, the dextrose being added to make the solution isotomic with blood.

If gastrointestinal secretions have been lost they should be replaced on a volume-for-volume basis with a mixed electrolyte solution of approximately the same composition as the fluid lost. Lactated Ringer's solution is usually adequate for such cases.

Abnormal losses of secretions occurring during therapy can be measured and replaced with lactated Ringer's solution as they occur.

In advanced cases of fluid and electrolyte depletion the signs of circulatory failure may be pronounced. In these cases it is advisable to expand the circulating blood volume before embarking on electrolyte replacement therapy. This can be achieved by transfusing plasma or a plasma substitute until the signs of circulatory failure regress. From a knowledge of the relative sizes of the body compartments it can be calculated that approximately 10% of the total fluid deficit may have to be replaced in this way. If a dehydrated animal requires emergency surgery the restoration of the normal circulating blood volume prior to anaesthesia is a matter of great importance.

Route of administration

The intravenous route is preferable whenever possible, but in certain circumstances venpuncture can be associated with considerable difficulties. In such cases the subcutaneous route of administration may have to be employed. The absorption of fluids given subcutaneously can be improved considerably by the addition of hyaluronidase.

Rate of transfusion

Clinical and experimental work has confirmed that electrolyte solutions can be safely transfused intravenously at a rate of 40 ml/kg body weight per hour. This represents 1 l/h for a 25 kg dog. This rate of transfusion has been sustained for several hours without untoward effects, but normal renal function is a necessary prerequisite. It is probably safer to start a transfusion more slowly until adequate urine production is established.

Monitoring

Following the institution of intravenous therapy it is important to monitor the total fluid intake (including fluids given by mouth) and also the total fluid output (especially urine output but also gastrointestinal secretions and uterine discharge). Information thus obtained is best recorded daily on a fluid chart and the balance then computed. Fluid charts are inevitably inaccurate as a result of technical difficulties in measurement, but they still provide a useful source of information.

Part C
Radiography

PETER WEBBON and CAROL FRANCE

Introduction

The object of radiography is to produce a diagnostically useful radiograph, or series of radiographs, of the appropriate part of the animal, correctly positioned, with optimum density, contrast and definition.

General considerations

The radiographic examination of the patient can be divided into several components, the interrelationship of which is summarized in Fig. 15.

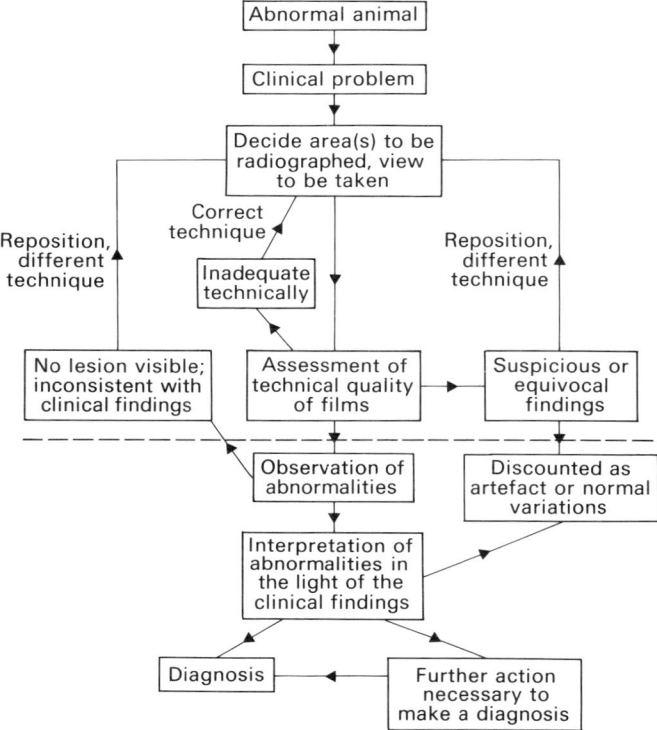

Fig. 15. A simple diagram to show some of the steps in a radiographic examination. The boxes above the broken line are concerned with the collection of information. Those below the broken line involve the assimilation and interpretation of the information. Errors made above the line cannot be corrected subsequently, so that mistakes in collecting the information may often be the limiting factor in a radiographic examination.

The clinical component

This consists of the recognition of a clinical problem, e.g. intermittent vomition, and the determination from the history and examination of the area of interest to be radiographed, e.g. the stomach. *The failure at this stage to decide on the correct radiographs to be taken will totally negate the value of the entire succeeding procedure.*

No amount of abdominal radiographs will reveal an oesophageal foreign body, neither will a poorly positioned view of the entire forelimb of a Labrador reveal the often subtle changes associated with elbow osteochondrosis.

Choice of exposure factors and ancillary equipment

The X-ray photons produced by a cheap portable machine are identical to those produced by the most expensive machine. The latter provides the potential to produce more X-ray photons in a shorter time and to achieve greater flexibility in the range of energy of the photons leaving the tube. It should therefore follow that, notwithstanding the limitations of portable equipment, a good radiographer should produce a top quality radiograph of all but the most difficult subjects. To blame one's X-ray machine for poor quality radiographs is as ridiculous as blaming a car for its driver's failure to read a map and reach a chosen destination (although the maximum speed of the car may be a factor in determining the journey time).

Positioning of the animal

The aim of positioning dogs for radiography must be to produce radiographs that can be compared with films of the same or other patients. This implies that standard procedures should be used. There will always be, however, occasions when extraordinary radiographic positions have to be invented to suit individual cases. Ideally, standard radiographic positions should be universally employed for all species. An inspection of the available texts on veterinary radiography will show that no such standardization has yet been attained, which means that it must be achieved within a particular practice.

Processing of the film

No single area of radiography is as crucial to the success of the entire procedure as the chemical processing of the film and especially its development. Only by standardizing film processing can any discussion of the choice of exposure factors be realistic. The basic rules to be obeyed are (any reader unwilling to obey these rules should proceed no further):

1 Use a heating system to maintain accurately and reliably the developer at the correct temperature (20°C).
2 Always develop the films for a fixed time (4 min) and do not rely on observing the degree of development by safelight.
3 Replenish the developer with the correct replenishing solution as necessary.

Assessment of the technical quality of the film

A poor quality film may fail to reveal a lesion or may lead to a misdiagnosis because of a technical artefact. It is the authors' experience that both heart size and pulmonary patterns are frequently thought to be abnormal by inexperienced radiologists on the basis of poor quality radiographs. It is not extending a healthy scepticism too far to assume that all lesions are artefacts or normal variations until proved otherwise by a logical consideration and elimination of the possible causes of the apparent lesion. It is at this stage that the decision should be taken to repeat any films which are inadequate and to correct any faults by recognizing their cause.

Observation of abnormalities

This requires both correct physical and psychological conditions. The physical requirements are a well-illuminated viewing box, a darkened room, a bright light source for darker areas of the film, and the minimum of distraction. With the exception of a viewing box few busy practitioners will realize the ideal conditions, especially the lack of distraction. On the basis of their experience of lesions missed in the activity of the X-ray room but seen easily in a more leisurely retrospective viewing, the authors would strongly recommend that a few minutes of each day should be devoted to a review of recent radiographs. The psychological requirements are theoretically as simple, but as difficult to achieve, and often reflect conflicts within the radiologist. A sceptical attitude to distinguish artefacts and normal variations from lesions has already been mentioned. This is, however, inevitably tempered by a desire to discover an explanation for the observed clinical signs, which may lead to over-reading of the films. It is also self-evident that it is easier to see the lesions which you expect to see. Whereas an inexperienced undergraduate is highly unlikely to notice an osteochrondritis dissecans lesion affecting the humeral head, an experienced radiologist will recognize it immediately. Such awareness and recognition of common syndromes must not lead to preconceptions which result in the radiologist overlooking unusual or unexpected changes.

Interpretation of the significance of any abnormalities observed.

This requires a sound knowledge of the spectrum of normality as well as a concept of pathology and how various pathological changes are reflected radiographically. With experience, intuition is also developed which is valuable in assessing the significance of a possible lesion. Many radiologists, when asked whether a suspect area on a film is or is not a lesion would answer that it does or not does 'look like one'. Their attempts lucidly to explain the reason behind their judgement would not be as successful as their intuition based on a vast subconscious store of visual images. There is no satisfactory alternative to experience in acquiring skill in radiology but the experience will only be valuable if reliable follow-ups as surgical findings, autopsies, biopsies or laboratory results are available.

The choice of exposure factors and ancillary equipment

The major variable factors under the radiographer's control are the kV (kilovolts), mA, (milliamps), s (exposure time,

sec), FFD (focus to film distance), the grid and the film/screen combination.

Kilovoltage

The energizing voltage of the X-ray tube is measured in kilovolts (kV). The energizing voltage controls the beam energy and also affects the number of X-ray photons which are produced. (Number, i.e. intensity of X-ray photons produced, is proportional to the square of the kV.)

As a general rule, keep in the high range when using low output equipment; the loss of contrast so produced is in practical terms scarcely noticed since kV changes only lead to very obvious contrast differences in the range 40–55 kV. However, when radiographing the extremities of small dogs using moderately fast intensifying screens, a low kV (i.e. 40–60) is necessary in conjunction with a low mAs. Some modern imported machines do not have a kV range which extends low enough so that slow intensifying screens, non-screen film, or a very long FFD must be used for this type of examination.

Milliamperage

The tube current is measured in milliamps (mA), and represents the number of electrons with which the target is bombarded. The number of X-ray photons is directly proportional to the mA. The tube current has no influence on the beam energy.

Timing

Exposure time is measured in seconds. Often combined with the mA as mAs. The intensity of the beam is proportional to the mAs. The beam energy is independent of it. The mA should be as high as possible to keep the exposure time as short as possible. In most portable machines the mA falls as the kV is increased and may not be variable by the radiographer.

Focus to film distance

This must be standardized and only altered under exceptional circumstances. For the average portable machine 75 cm is probably the best compromise between geometric distortion and high exposures.

Grid

Whether or not to use a grid, and the type to use. The use of a grid is extremely important, second only to correct development in obtaining high contrast radiographs of the thicker parts (chest, abdomen, pelvis) of large dogs. The initial cost is not a valid reason for not using a grid. The necessity to increase the exposure factors by two to three times may be a limiting factor when radiographing potentially moving parts (thorax and to a lesser degree the abdomen) if this requires an increase in exposure time. For stationary subjects, of which the pelvis of an anaesthetised dog is an obvious example, an exposure time well in excess of 1 sec can be used to accommodate a grid.

The film/screen combination

It is in this area that most technical progress has been recently made. Several phosphors are now used in intensifying screens in addition to calcium tungstate, e.g. lead, strontium barium sulphate and activated oxysulphides or oxybromides of lanthanum or gadolinium (the 'rare earth' phosphors). Whatever phosphor is used a range of screen speeds will generally be available and the range may be further expanded by using a different film. For example, the 3M Trimax range of intensifying screens provides four screen speeds (Alpha 2, 4, 8 and 16), which can be used with four film types (XUD, XD, XM and latitude film). By the intelligent use of new imaging systems most practices could improve the standard of their radiography. No two practices will be alike and before purchasing new equipment most would do well to take advice from an independent radiologist. The aim is to have screens and films which are simple to use and enable the potential of any X-ray machine to be achieved. This will probably mean a fast screen/film combination for use with low output equipment but a slower system giving excellent detail and contrast if a more powerful unit is to be used.

The application of exposure factors

Due to a variety of reasons, especially the age of the X-ray tube and the type of voltage rectification which is incorporated into the machine, exposure factors are applicable only to the unit for which they are intended. However, a good guide to correct exposure factors can be obtained from published lists.

Within a practice it is essential to have an exposure record or chart to maintain the consistency of X-ray examinations (when, for example, assessing the progression of a lesion) and to enable newcomers to use the equipment. It cannot be overstressed that all these considerations are irrelevant unless processing is standardized.

Two methods are available to choose exposure factors. The first depends on adequate records of each exposure, the size and breed of the patient and comments on the quality of the film. When a reasonable number of exposures have been recorded it is then easy to look back through the records for a similar animal of the type to be radiographed. Alternatively an exposure chart can be constructed from the records for small, large, medium and giant dogs.

The second type of exposure chart involves measuring the part to be radiographed and calculating the exposure on this basis. This system has the advantage that once one reasonable film has been taken with a new unit, it should be possible to calculate the exposure for any part of any other animal. One method of devising an exposure chart based on measurement is described by Morgan, Silverman & Zontine (1977).

Take a medium-sized dog and radiograph its abdomen in a lateral projection using 70 kV and varying mAs until a good radiograph is obtained. The mAs setting should be doubled each time, e.g. 2, 4 and 8 mAs, until by trial and error the correct setting is obtained. Measure the abdomen in cm at its largest point. When radiographing other dogs, for each additional centimetre in thickness (providing the mAs remains constant) add 2 kV up to 80 kV and 3 kV above 80 kV. The kV is reduced similarly for smaller abdomens. This means it is possible, provided all else is kept constant, to construct an exposure chart for dogs' abdomens of all sizes.

The same chart can be applied to other parts of the body and other animals by applying simple rules (although it is easier to construct charts for other anatomical areas).
1   Halve mAs for puppies and cats.
2   Double mAs for heavily muscled or fat dogs, or plaster cast.
3   Increase kV by 5–10 for areas composed largely of bone (skull, pelvis).
4   Increase kV by 10–15 if a grid is to be used.
5   Decrease kV by 5–10 for soft tissue radiographs, e.g. of the neck.

The exposure factors thus obtained will still need to be modified in some cases, for example to keep the time short for chest radiographs.

The manipulation of exposure factors

It is sometimes necessary to convert exposure factors from those in published lists to those suitable for the equipment to be used.

An example of why this may be necessary and how it should be carried out will illustrate the underlying principles.

Let us suppose that you have purchased a 30/110 portable X-ray unit (which produces 10 mA at 110 kV, 15 mA at 100 kV, 25 mA at 85 kV and 30 mA at 70 kV), and that your list of exposure factors is for a 20 mA portable machine with kV range of 40–90. Your first patient for radiography may be a 20 kg Collie with a painful elbow. The exposure data for an elbow of a dog of this size quoted on your list are:

AP   60 kV 0.20 sec
Lat.   60 kV 0.10 sec

These factors are for a 75 cm FFD, operating at 20 mA using standard screens and medium speed film. To calculate the new exposure factors for the AP projection:
Step 1. Calculate the mAs; mA × 0.20 (i.e. 20 × 0.20) = 4 mAs.
Step 2. Select the nearest kV to the suggested kV setting; 70 kV is the nearest to 60 (one of the disadvantages of the machine used in this example is the limited kV range).
Step 3. Correct the mAs for the new kV setting; as a

practical rule, increasing the kV by 10 will necessitate halving the mAs and vice versa; thus the new mAs should be 2.

Step 4. Calculate the new exposure time; s = mAs/mA; s = 2/30 (since at 70 kV the machine produced 30 mA) = 0.07 sec.

The same calculation can be carried out for the lateral view to produce a new exposure of 0.03 sec (all of the exposure times are approximate and may have to be altered a little to coincide with an exposure setting on the machine).

Further compensation will have to be made if a longer or shorter FFD than 75 cm is used and if the screen/film combination is faster or slower than the standard screen and medium film quoted in the table.

FFD correction. X-rays obey the inverse square law so that for the lateral view in the example, if a 1 m FFD is to be used:

$$\frac{new\ s}{0.03} = \frac{100^2}{75^2}$$
$$New\ s = 0.05.$$

The conversion factor to compensate for different films and screens has to be worked out by trial and error, but provided that the same combination is always used it will remain constant throughout all examinations.

A further example will illustrate the benefits obtained from manipulating the exposure factors.

Subject. 40 kg Labrador with a clinical diagnosis of hydrothorax. Exposure for 20 mA portable:

DV   90 kV 0.16 sec.
Lat.   80 kV 0.10 sec.

75 cm FFD standard screen, medium film, 20 mA.

This exposure would almost certainly be too low if the clinical diagnosis of hydrothorax is correct since much of the air in the lungs will be replaced by free fluid. It will therefore be necessary at least to double the exposures given.

Step 1. Calculate the mAs; DV—20×0.16 = 3.2; Lat. —20×0.10 = 2.0; double the mAs because of the dog's clinical problem. DV 6.4; Lat. 4.0.

Step 2. Select the nearest kV setting to the suggested exposure. Since the dog is dyspnoeic it will be advantageous in this case to use a high kV and to keep the exposure time as short as possible.

Step 3. Correct the mAs for the new kV setting. By applying the practical rule of 10 (kV + by 10 ≡ doubling the mAs) a table of mAs values and exposure times can be constructed for each of the kV/mA settings on the 30/110 machine.

Table 1 suggests that the optimum kV setting for both examinations is probably 100 kV (or possibly 110 kV for the DV view). It should also be noted that effective freezing of respiratory and cardiac movement requires an exposure time of 0.03 s or less in a dog breathing normally.

If the thoracic spine, rather than the lungs, was the area of interest, it would be better to use a lower kV to enhance bone/soft tissue contrast and to employ a grid for the same

purpose. Both would lead to a considerable increase in exposure time.

Table 1.

kV	mA	mAs		s	
		DV	Lat.	DV	Lat.
70	30	25.6	8.0	0.8	0.3
85	25	9.6	3.0	0.4	0.12
100	15	3.2	1.0	0.2	0.06
110	10	1.6	0.5	0.16	0.05

Processing the film

It cannot be reiterated too frequently nor too strongly that correct chemical processing is the key to a general improvement of radiographic standards.

Chemical processing consists, under most circumstances, of: (a) develop; (b) rinse; (c) fix; (d) wash; (e) dry. The cycle may be carried out manually or automatically.

Manual processing

Development

The principle of development is that those molecules of silver bromide which have been exposed to light or X-ray energy are reduced to black metallic silver, while most of the unexposed crystals are not reduced. The developer solution must, therefore, be selective in reducing only exposed crystals, and to obtain optimum image quality all of the exposed crystals need to be reduced. These aims are largely realized by modern developers *provided that they are used as directed.*

Four factors are critical: (a) Time of development; (b) temperature of solution: (c) agitation during development; (d) age and exhaustion of solution.

Time of development

Development for too short a period produces low film density (too few silver bromide crystals reduced) and poor contrast (Fig. 16a). If the film is left in the developer for too long the solution loses its selective nature and reduces unexposed crystals, thus increasing the level of background 'fog' (Fig. 16b). From Fig. 16b it can clearly be seen that developing the film for less than 3–4 min will inevitably result in poor contrast. To ensure optimum image quality, all films must be developed for 4 min (at 20°C).

Temperature of developer

Within a short range (18–24°C) it is theoretically possible to alter development time to compensate for temperature

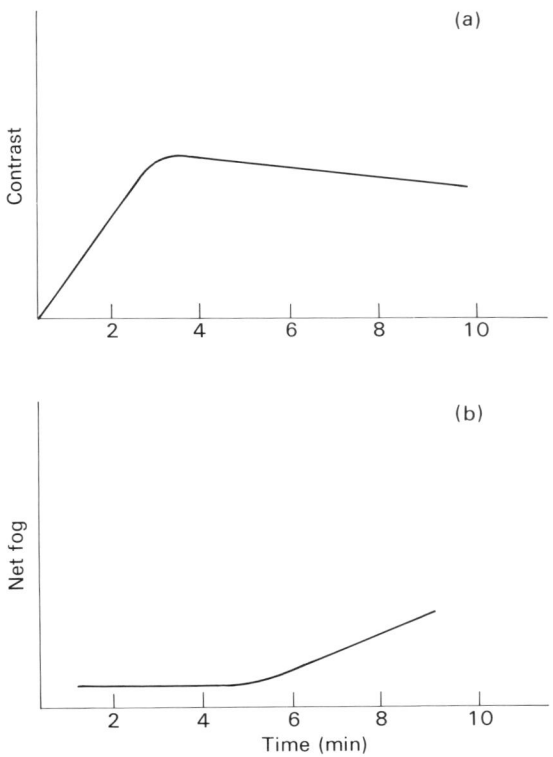

Fig. 16. Effects of the development time on relative contrast and net fog.

variations and to produce satisfactory radiographs. In practice this leads to difficulty. The developer temperature must be maintained at 20°C either by a thermostatically controlled water bath or more simply by a fish tank heater.

Agitation during development

During the 4-min period the film should be agitated for the first few seconds after immersion and thereafter for 5 sec every minute.

Exhaustion of developer

During normal use, chemical and physical changes occur, both of which are exaggerated by accidental overheating.
Chemical changes: developing agents are oxidized; pH falls; concentration of bromide ions increases.
Physical changes: volume of developer decreases due to carry over on the wet film and evaporation of water; concentration of the preservative decreases.

Because these changes occur the developer must be changed frequently or replenished. Very few practices use developer replenisher yet its use is one of the most important factors in consistently obtaining high quality radiographs. The instructions for the use of replenisher are complicated, based on the amount of films processed. In general, it is adequate to mark the developer level and to top this up with replenisher solution as necessary, provided that most of the loss of developer is due to use and not to dehydration.

If a practice takes only a small number of radiographs per week it is worthwhile considering the use of a dish rather than tank technique. The procedure requires that about 1–2 l developer (or less) are made up at one time (the cost is approximately that of one sheet of 30×40 cm X-ray film). The temperature can easily be controlled by the temperature of the water in which the solution is made. The radiographs are then developed in a shallow photographic dish (or clean washing-up bowl) and by choosing to carry out all elective radiography on 1 day/week the increased cost is negligible. Any practice which is in doubt about the improvement in image quality produced by the consistent use of dish developer should try it. Those practices which have a higher radiographic work load and use a developer tank *must* use replenisher.

1 *Rinsing*. This should be for 15 sec in running water.
2 *Fixation*. The fixing bath: (a) arrests development; (b) removes undeveloped silver halide ('clears' the film); (c) 'fixes' the image to make it permanent; (d) hardens the gelatin in the emulsion.

Fixing time. 5–10 min.

Temperature of solution. Not as critical as for the developer, but preferably within 5°C of the developer temperature.

Exhaustion of the fixer and silver recovery. Soluble silver crystals build up in the fixer until it can no longer function efficiently. At this stage the fixer should be changed and it makes good financial and environmental sense that the silver is recovered. This service is provided by a number of specialist companies who will collect the exhausted fixer and will also purchase scrapped or old X-ray film.

3 *Washing*. This needs to be for 10 min in running (i.e. changed at least four times) water. Washing should be performed as soon as possible after fixation and the film not allowed to partially dry first.

4 *Drying*. This is usually in air. Hang the film by a clip, not in a channel hanger. Drying marks (due to water streaking the film) will occur unless the films are immersed in a wetting agent before drying.

Automatic processing

Using this technique the entire process occurs in a single unit at a higher temperature than for manual processing. The processor may fit on a table top or be larger and self-standing. Any busy small animal practice would be well advised to consider automatic processing, due to the time it saves (the cycle may be as short as 90 s), the consistency of the processing (the chemicals are constantly replenished), and the finished film which is dry for viewing.

Assessment of the technical quality of the film

The following need to be checked to assess the technical quality of an X-ray film:

1 *Density*. The degree to which the film is blackened. It can be measured by the light transmission through the film.

2 *Contrast*. The difference in density between two parts of film. A high contrast film is black and white; a low contrast film is composed of shades of grey.

3 *Definition*. The amount of fine detail that can be perceived on the film. A 'sharp' film has good definition.

4 *Marks*. There should be an absence of extraneous marks and discolorations.

5 *Collimation*. The beam should be centred on the area of interest and no larger than necessary.

6 *Identification*. Correct marking of the film to identify the animal and date of radiography.

7 *Positioning*. Correct positioning of the animal.

Table 2. The common causes of poor radiographic image quality

Low contrast	Underdevelopment
	Scatter fog
Density	
Too dark	Over exposure
	Incorrect safelight
	Light leaks in dark room
	Fogging due to overdevelopment
Too light	Underdevelopment
	Underexposure
Lack of definition (blurring)	Movement of animal
	Movement of X-ray machine

Table 3.

The criteria of good radiographic quality control	Variable factors under radiographer's control
Correct film density	Development
	Exposure factors
	Darkroom (safelight filter and bulb and blackout)
Good contrast	Development
	Use of a grid
	Use of intensifying screens
	Beam collimation
	Beam energy
Good definition	Short exposure time
	Patient restraint
	Tube head must be stationary
Adequate collimation	Cone or variable diaphragm collimator
Accurate identification	Lead letters, radiodense tape, or photographic marker
Correct positioning	Position of animal
	Direction of beam
	Patient restraint

The common causes of poor radiographic image quality and the variable factors which control the image are shown in Tables 2 and 3. A procedure to diagnose and correct common faults is discussed in the following section.

If the development procedure within a practice is correct, all other aspects of radiography will rapidly follow.

Fault finding in poor radiographs

Look at the background (on a viewing box only a poorly visible shadow of your finger or a pen should be seen through the background). Background will be (a) too light (i.e. grey), or (b) correct density (you are unlikely to decide subjectively that it is too dark).

Background too light

The film is *probably* underdeveloped. It *may* be underexposed due to:

1 Poor exposure factor choice.

2 Reduced line voltage to machine.

3 Very small or poorly calcified subject requiring very low exposure, thus producing a grey background.

To decide whether underdeveloped/underexposed:

1 Look at the image. If it is only a silhouette of the subject the film is underexposed or correctly exposed and underdeveloped. If the image is well penetrated the film is overexposed and underdeveloped.

2 Develop a second film, same subject and exposure factors, using the dish technique (see earlier) and fresh developer:

(a) *Background black, good image*. Alter development technique by using dish technique or replenisher. Keep exposure factors as before.

(b) *Background black, image too dark*. Original film was overexposed then underdeveloped. Alter development technique and reduce exposure factors by at least 50%.

(c) *Background still grey*. Original fault was underexposure. If this has just occurred check first the input voltage to the machine.

Background has or appears to have correct density

Look at the image:

1 Too black may be overexposed or fogged. To decide, look at any part of the film which should not have been exposed to X-rays. If this is clear the problem was overexposure; if grey the film is fogged. Causes of fogging producing dark image in descending order of importance:

a) safelight filter cracked or bulb too bright;

b) minor white light leak in darkroom;

c) old film or film exposed to secondary radiation or chemicals;

d) overdevelopment.

2 Low contrast (the commonest cause of low contrast is underdevelopment, but this will produce a grey back-

ground). Second commonest cause of poor contrast is scatter fog. To reduce scatter collimate the beam, and use a grid. kV affects contrast but only significantly in the low (i.e. 40–60) range.

3 Image blurred. In practice due to movement of either the patient or the tube head.

4 Film is discoloured (usually yellow/brown) after storage, sometimes with crystalline deposits. Due to poor fixation/washing. Change the fixer (remember silver recovery) and ensure that the wash water is changed at least 4 times in the 10 min for which the film should be washed.

5 White marks on the radiograph. Dirt on the intensifying screens. These need to be cleaned regularly with soap and water or screen cleaning fluid.

There are many other, less common, causes of poor radiographs. However, attention to those listed above will correct a large majority of the faults encountered in practical radiography.

Positioning for radiography

It is most convenient to describe the relationship of the primary beam to the animal with reference to the latter in a normal standing position:

1 For trunk and spine, the dorso-ventral (DV) or ventro-dorsal (VD).

2 For limbs, the antero-posterior (AP) or postero-anterior (PA).

3 Recumbent lateral (left or right depending on the side on which the dog lies).

4 For limbs, the latero-medial (LM) or medio-lateral (ML).

Oblique views of limbs should be described with reference to the path of the beam, e.g. antero-postero-medio-lateral oblique (APMLO).

For the skull, several projections may be used:

DV.

VD.

DV or VD intra-oral using non-screen film.

Open mouth AP.

Frontal sinus AP.

Basilar view for foramen magnum and cranial vault.

Oblique view for teeth, temporomandibular joints and tympanic bullae.

Several textbooks illustrate positions for canine radiography (see Further Reading, p. 181) and vary considerably in their approach to the various anatomical areas.

Most important of all is that each practice, within the constraints imposed by clinical considerations and the safety of the radiographer, should adhere to a strict routine and a standard procedure. This is the only way in which experience can be developed and comparable films obtained for all patients.

There are fundamental principles related to patient restraint and accurate positioning which should always be borne in mind.

Patient restraint

General anaesthesia, sedation and positioning aids should always be used in preference to manual restraint. The exceptions to this rule, based on clinical grounds only, are few. Convenience and speed are not acceptable reasons for exposing personnel to the potential hazard of ionizing radiation. There are good reasons in addition to safety for the use of restraint other than by assistants. These include:

1 Greater patient comfort, especially where the indication for radiography is painful, e.g. fractures, disc protrusions, painful arthropathies, when accurate positioning would exacerbate the pain and a poorly positioned radiograph may not be of diagnostic quality.

2 Better and easier reproducibility of standard positions in all patients, especially those with widely different conformation.

3 If a film tray is used, frequently in conjunction with a moving grid, the position of the animal can be maintained during processing of the film. Any alterations in position can then be made with reference to the processed radiograph. This is of particular value in skull and pelvic radiography.

4 With a little forethought one anaesthetic can be used for diagnosis and treatment or several diagnostic procedures. For example, there is little point in struggling with a distressed dog to produce a radiograph of a femoral fracture if the dog will subsequently be anaesthetised to repair the injury. Similarly, a dog with chronic broncho-pulmonary disease requiring endoscopy is conveniently radiographed at the same time.

5 The use of a general anaesthetic abolishes the subjective (and possibly minimizes the objective) side effects of injected contrast media.

General guidelines

With a few exceptions, all films should be exposed with the area of interest parallel to the film in two planes, in the centre of the primary beam and at right angles to it.

For lateral projections of the trunk and axial skeleton most dogs will need some support to keep the trunk parallel to the film. This padding will be minimal in very narrow dogs like Salukis, but extensive in dogs with large thoraxes and narrow pelvises like Staffordshire Bull Terriers. Foam pads should support the chin and nose, the mid-cervical and lumbar spine and the sternum. The upper limbs are supported by sand bags and both fore and hind limbs are extended away from the trunk by sand bags or ties. For lateral projection of the limbs foam pads will be needed to ensure true lateral views. For example, to produce a medio-lateral view of the stifle the hock must be elevated, thus rotating the stifle outwards so that it lies parallel to the film.

For VD and DV views foam trunk supports are especially valuable. The entire animal should be symmetrically postioned since experience will show that it is, for example, very difficult to produce a straight pelvis film if the head, neck and forelimbs are not symmetrically positioned.

These general principles and the use of positioning aids are illustrated in the following sections.

Skull

Lateral skull (Fig. 17)

Place a foam wedge under the jaw to bring the sagittal plane parallel to the film.

Long thin-necked dogs, e.g. Dobermanns, need a sand-bag under the neck to bring the head into true lateral position.

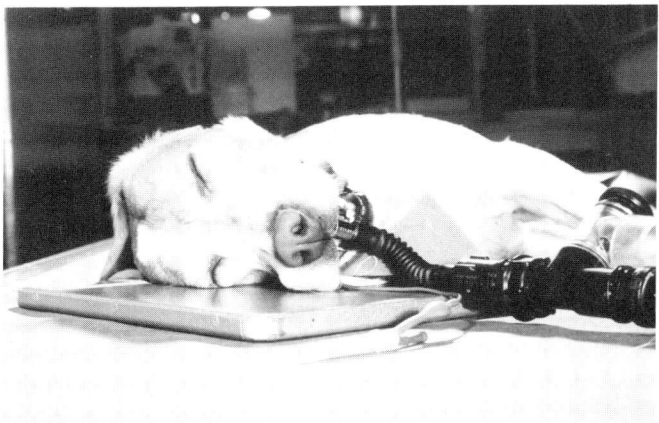

Fig. 17.

Dorso-ventral intra-oral skull (Figs 18 and 19)

Non-screen film is introduced, corner first, into the mouth so that more of the nasal cavity is visualized. Avoid pulling the film across the points of the canine teeth—this will leave black marks on the film. (A VD intra-oral film is very useful for examining the mandible.)

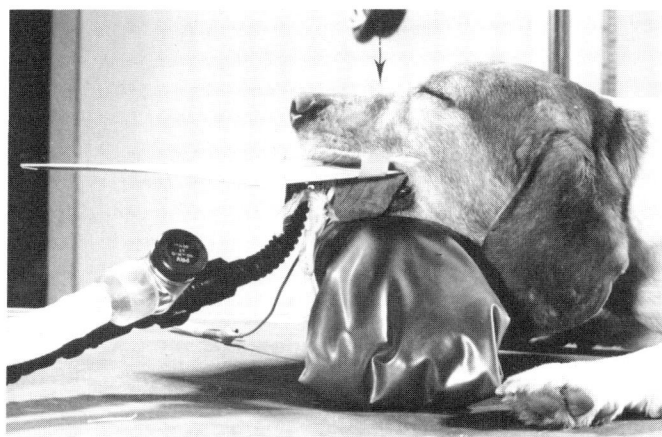

Fig. 18.

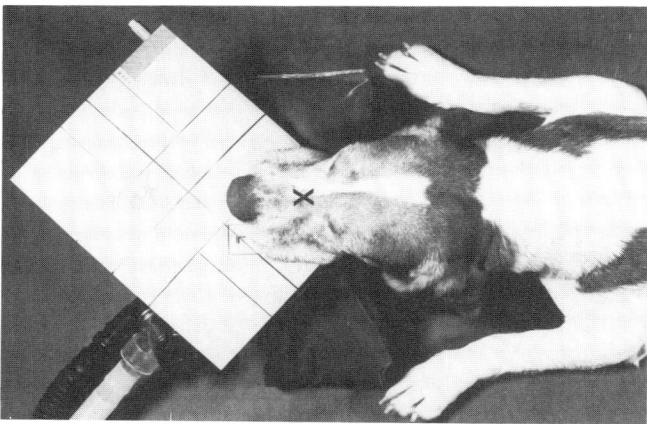

Fig. 19.

Antero-posterior skull (Figs 20 and 21)

1 For tympanic bullae. The dog is placed in dorsal recumbency and the position is maintained with foam pads and sandbags. Ties are put behind the upper and lower canines, the nose and jaw are pulled down to approximately 45° from perpendicular. Pull the tongue well out of the way as this can give false densities on the X-ray. Remove endotracheal tube and centre 5° to feet.

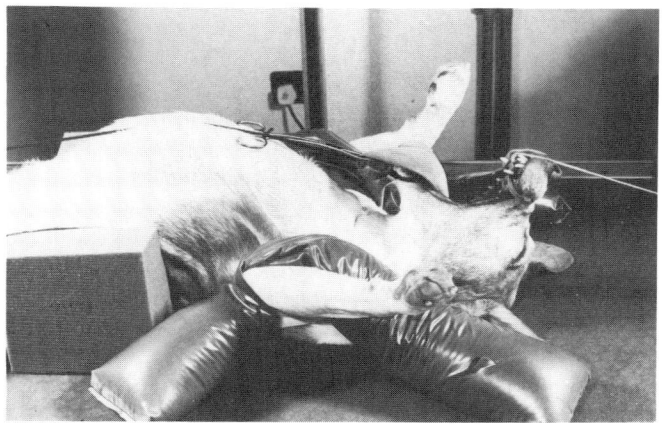

Fig. 20.

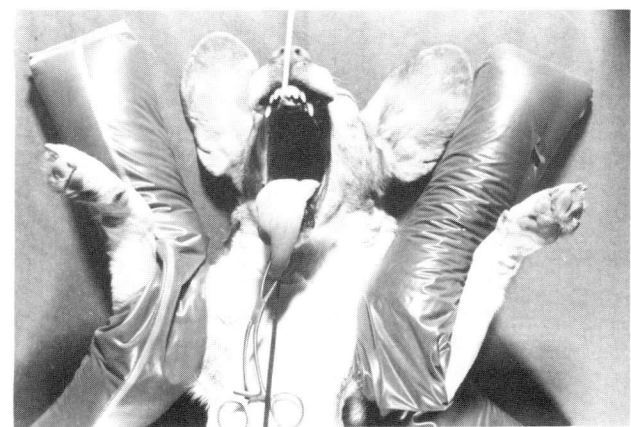

Fig. 21.

2 For odontoid peg. The nose is maintained in a perpendicular position to the cassette and the mandible pulled down. Use a straight tube and centre straight through open mouth.

3 For frontal sinuses. The nose is perpendicular to the cassette and the central ray goes through the centre of the frontal sinuses.

4 For foramen magnum. Put a tie around the nose and pull towards the chest to approximately 10°. The tube is angled 15–30° to feet and centre between the eyes.

Open mouth view—nares (Figs 22, 23 and 24)

The dog is placed in dorsal recumbency in foam cutouts, and supported on either side by sandbags draped over the front legs. A sandbag is placed under the neck to bring the hard palate parallel to the film. Use a mouth gag to open the mouth as much as possible and tongue foreps to pull the tongue right out of the way. Remove the endotracheal tube, angle the tube 8–10° to feet.

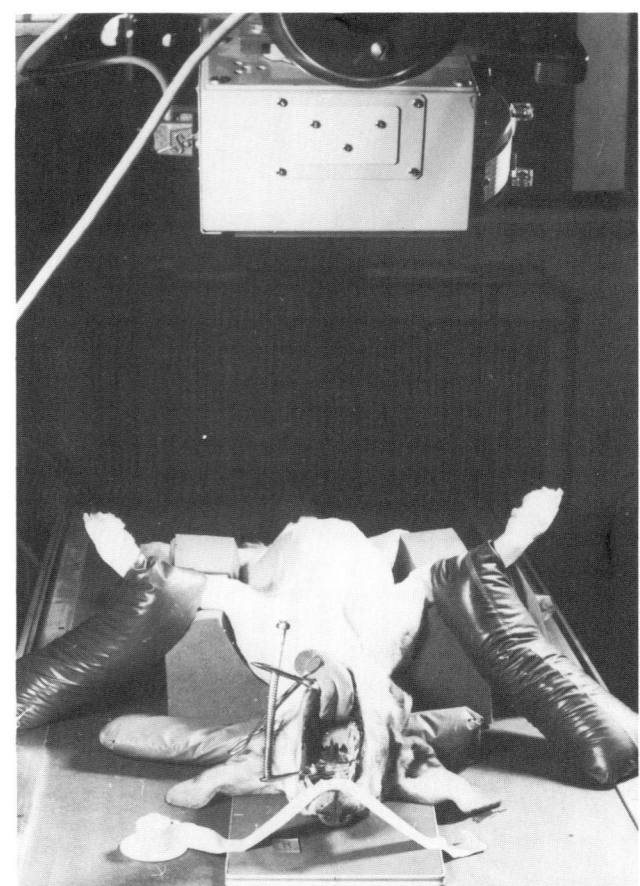

Fig. 23.

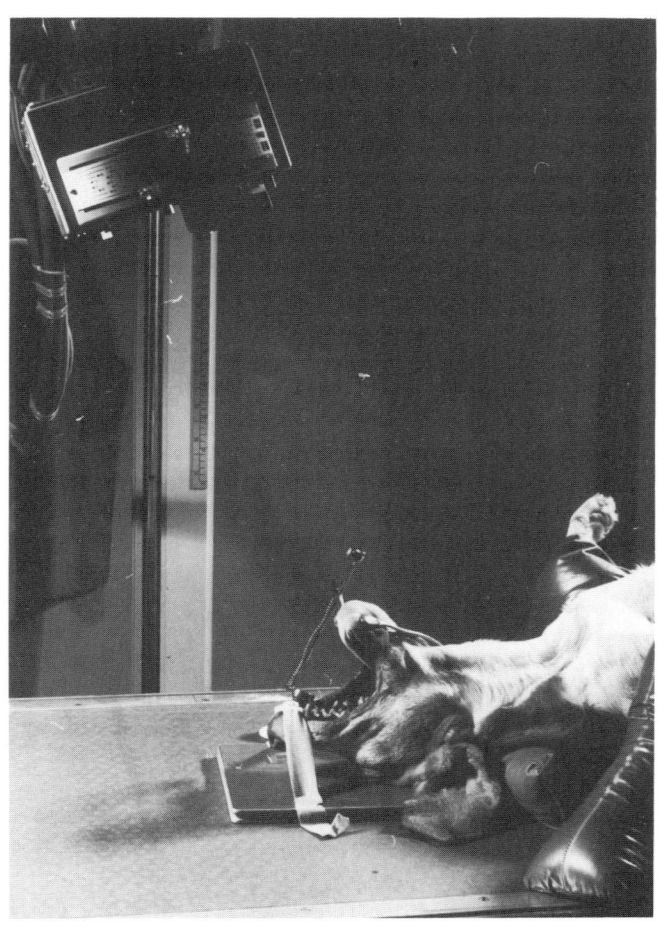

Fig. 22.

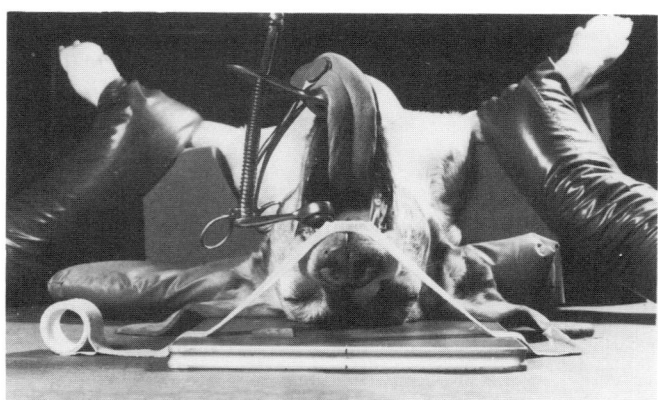

Fig. 24.

Thorax and abdomen

Lateral thorax (Figs 25 and 26)

Right lateral recumbency. The front legs are extended forward with ties in the anaesthetized dog and sandbags in the conscious animal. In the conscious dog a sandbag is placed over the extended neck. The hindlegs are held in extension with sandbags; one on the lower leg and another over the upper leg. A foam wedge may be useful between the stifles, especially in the conscious dog. In deep-chested dogs a foam wedge is required below the sternum to prevent rotation.

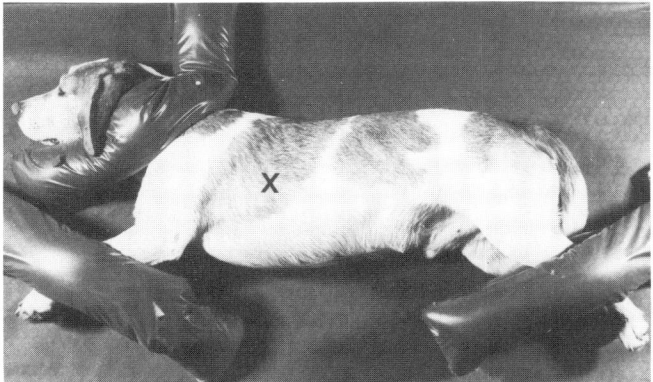

Fig. 25.

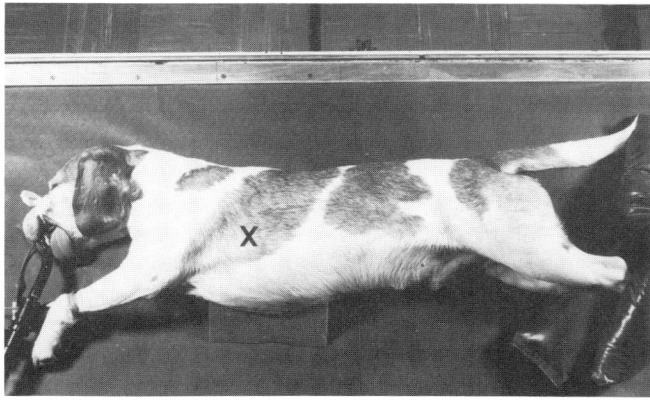

Fig. 26.

Ventro-dorsal thorax (for lung fields) (Fig. 27)

To achieve dorsal recumbency, place a foam support below the neck and one under the lumbar region. Extend the limbs and hold in position with sandbags. Make sure that the rib cage is straight and that the entire dog is symmetricaly positioned.

The exposure is made on full inspiration. (In the anaesthetized dog the lung fields should be inflated several times before the exposure.)

Since all exposures of the lungs are made on full inspiration, a short time is needed. If high output is available an increase in focus–film distance will prevent magnification distortion.

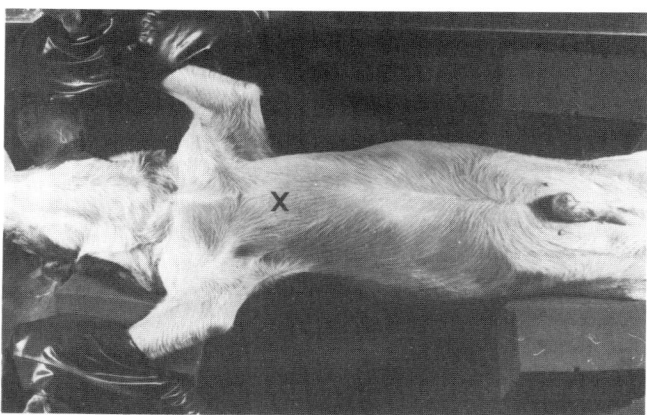

Fig. 27.

Dorso-ventral thorax (for heart) (Fig. 28)

The dog is in sternal recumbency with forelimbs extended forward and held by sandbags. The dog's head rests on these pads and a sandbag is draped over the neck. The hindlegs are set square in normal position and sandbags placed on either side. Make sure the rib cage is straight. In the anaesthetized animal the forelegs are pulled further forward and held in place by sandbags behind the elbows.

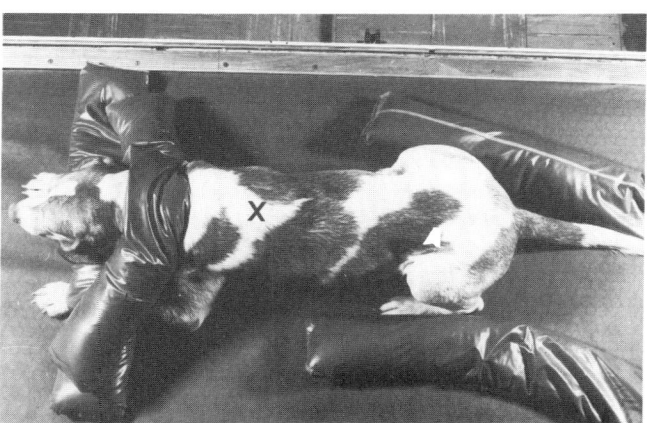

Fig. 28.

Lateral abdomen (Fig. 29)

Right or left recumbency will be determined by the indication for radiography.

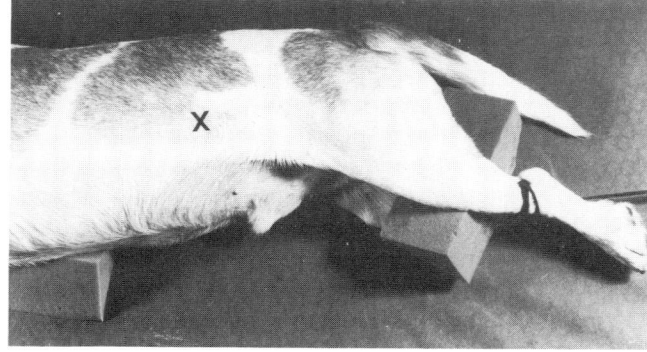

Fig. 29.

The hindlegs are drawn back to eliminate soft tissue density over the bladder region and held in place by sandbags or a tie. Pull the front legs forward and put a foam wedge under the sternum and between the stifles bringing the whole body lateral to the table top. Centre mid abdomen.

Ventro-dorsal abdomen (Fig. 30)

The dog in dorsal recumbency with a foam cutout under the thorax and sandbags over all the limbs. Make sure the animal is straight and centre mid abdomen.

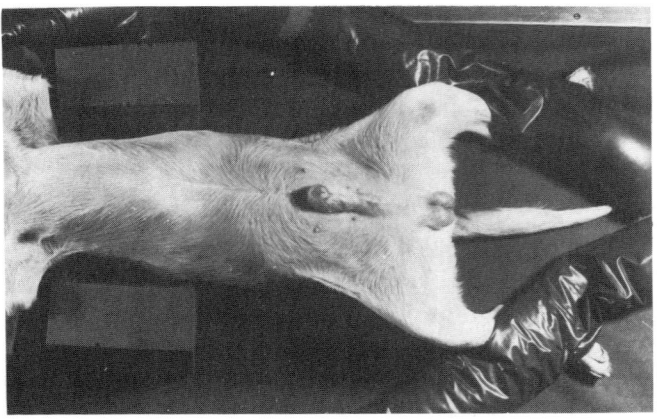

Fig. 30.

Spine and pelvis

Ventro-dorsal cervical, thoracic and lumbar spine (Fig. 31)

The dog is placed in dorsal recumbency in foam cutouts and sandbags for support and the forelegs are pulled down by means of ties or draped with sandbags, and a sandbag may be placed over the jaw. In long thin-necked dogs a bag is needed under the mid cervical spine to prevent it from dipping.

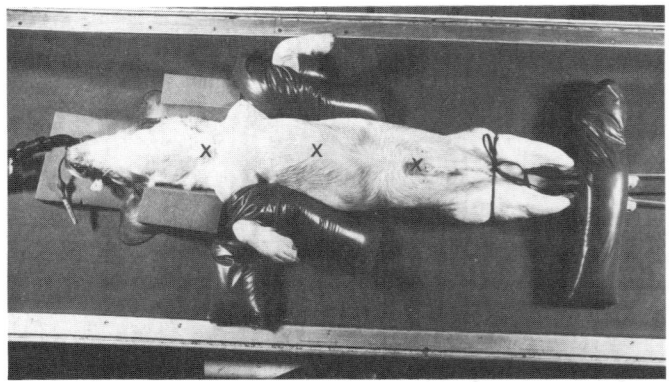

Fig. 31.

Lateral thoracic and lumbar spine, and lateral pelvis (Fig. 32)

The dog is in lateral recumbency with the front legs pulled forward and hindlegs pulled back by means of ties. Place a foam wedge under the sternum to prevent the thorax from dipping and a small wedge is needed between the stifles to bring the pelvis into a lateral position.

For thoracic spine centre through T6, for the lumbar spine centre L3, and for the pelvis centre through the acetabulum. For pelvic radiography the affected side should be closer to the film.

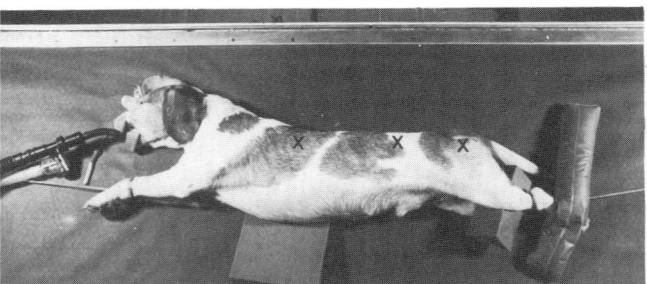

Fig. 32.

Lateral cervical spine (Figs 33 and 34)

The dog is placed in lateral recumbency. A tie on the upper limbs pulls them back to eliminate superimposition at the cervico-thoracic junction. A foam wedge is placed under the jaw to bring the head into true lateral position and a pad is also used in the mid cervical region to prevent the spine from dipping.

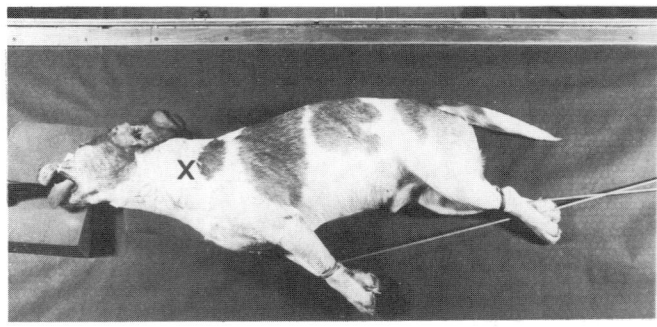

Fig. 33.

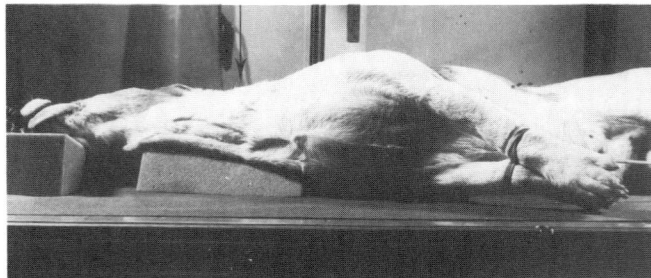

Fig. 34.

Ventro-dorsal pelvis (Fig. 35)

Place the dog in dorsal recumbency with a foam cutout under the mid thorax and sandbags over the front legs. Ties are put above the hocks and hindlegs are extended and tied to the end of a table—a small sandbag is placed under the feet and the legs are internally rotated and a tie placed just above both stifles. A sandbag is then placed over the feet to keep the limbs equidistant from the table top.

Centre through the acetabulum, making sure the iliac crests and top of the stifle joints are included for HD scheme. Right and left letters should be placed on the film and collimate.

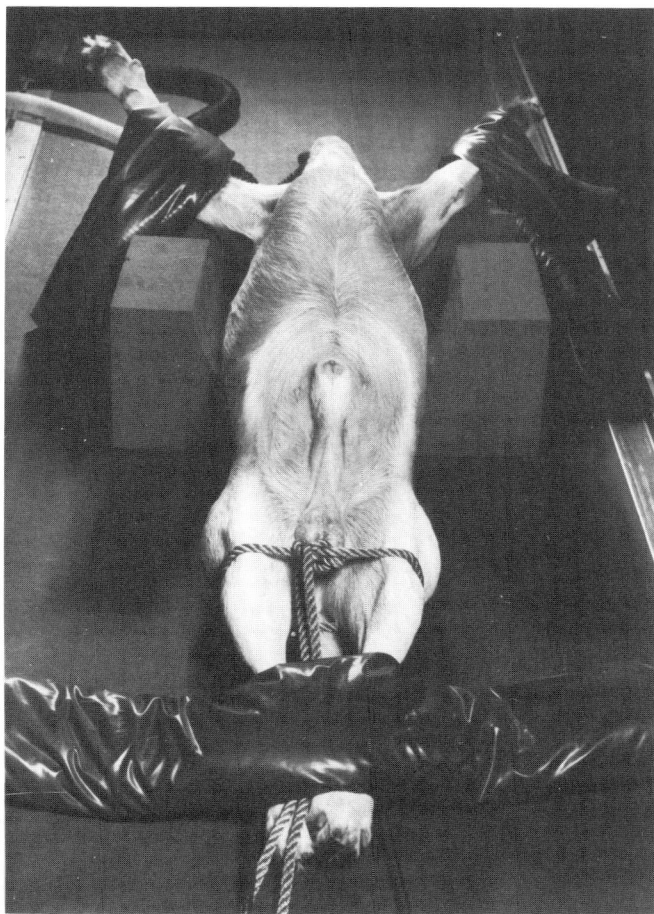

Fig. 35.

Foreleg and hindleg

Lateral foreleg (Figs 36 and 37)

Place the dog on the affected side. The upper leg is pulled out of the way with a tie and the affected limb is placed in the lateral position with foam pads under the elbow or carpus depending on site of X-ray.

For the shoulder the neck is extended with a sandbag and the lower limb pulled downward and forward with a tie to avoid superimposition of the trachea on the joint.

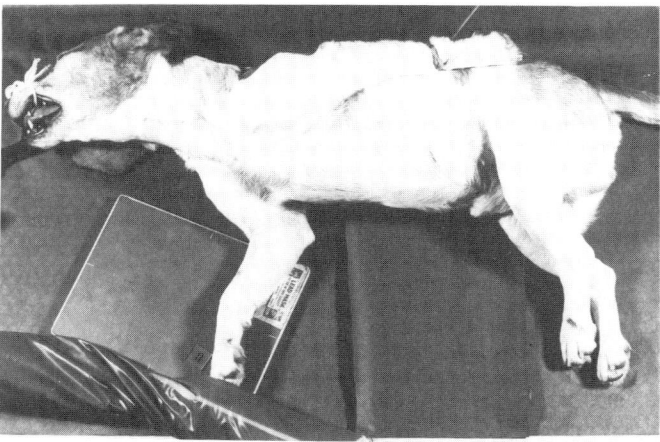

Fig. 36.

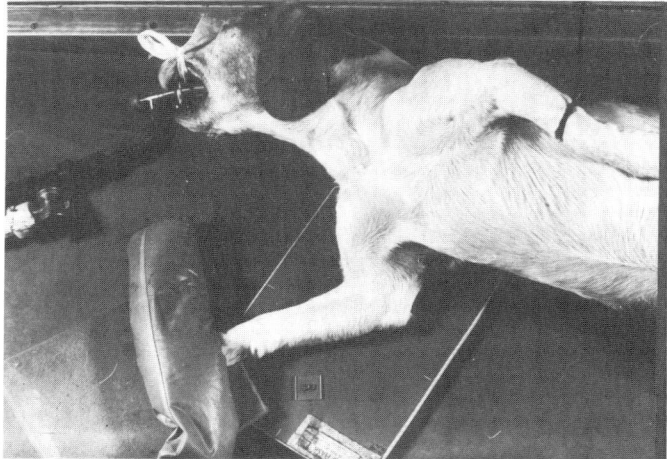

Fig. 37.

Postero-anterior foreleg (Fig. 38)

The dog is supported in dorsal recumbency with a foam pad and sandbags. The limb is extended with a tie and depressed with a sandbag. Deflect the head away from the affected limb.

This position is suitable for the elbow, humerus, shoulder joint and scapula.

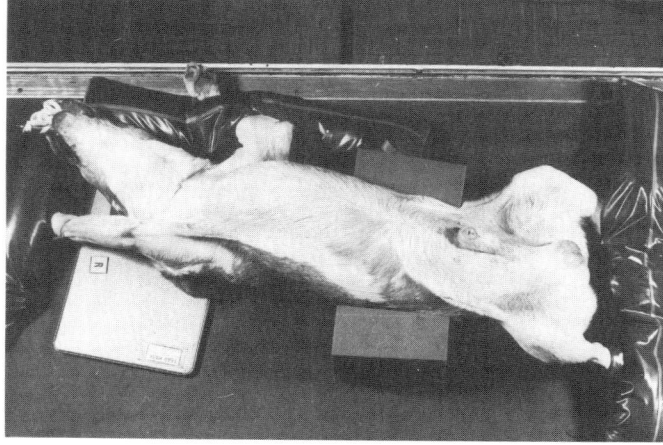

Fig. 38.

Antero-posterior foreleg (Figs 39 and 40)

In sternal recumbency with a sandbag under the unaffected limb and head pulled to that side. The affected limb is extended and a sandbag placed behind the elbow and along the side of the body. If the elbow is required the head is supported on a larger wedge and pulled as far over as possible to eliminate soft tissue density; the angle of the tube can also be altered.

For the shoulder joint a PA view is required.

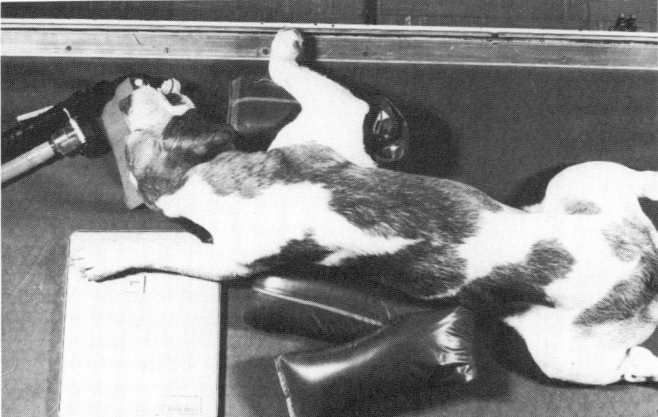

Fig. 39.

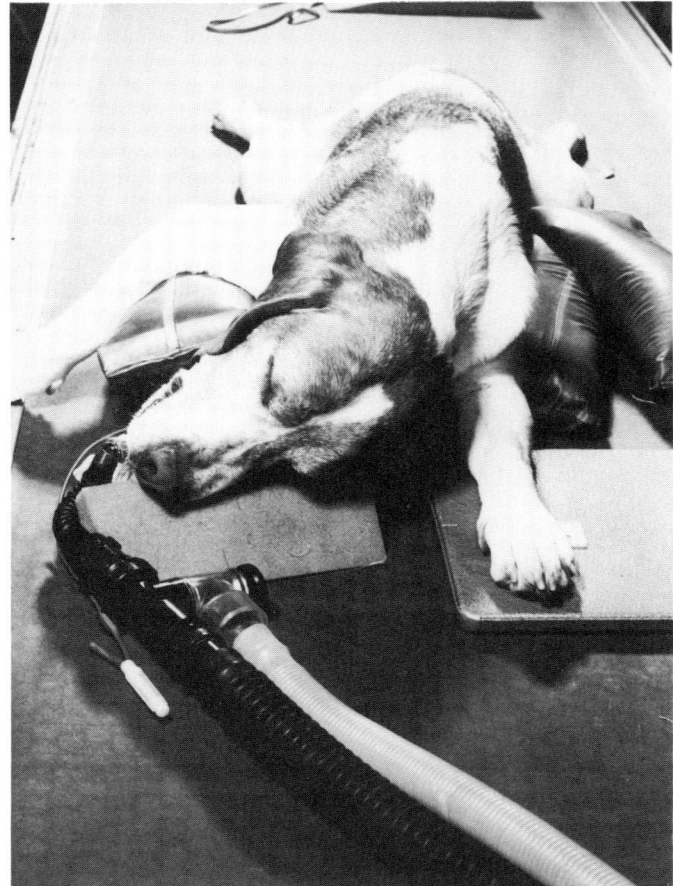

Fig. 40.

Lateral hindleg (Fig. 41)

The animal is in lateral recumbency with the affected side down. The unaffected leg is pulled out of the way by means of a tie, and the required area is placed over the cassette. Foam wedges can be used under the foot or stifle to bring the limb parallel to the film.

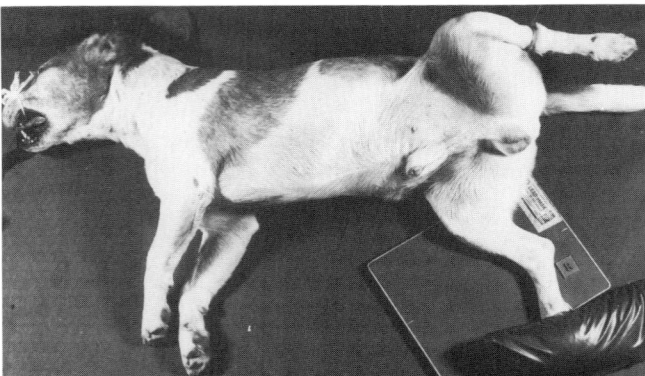

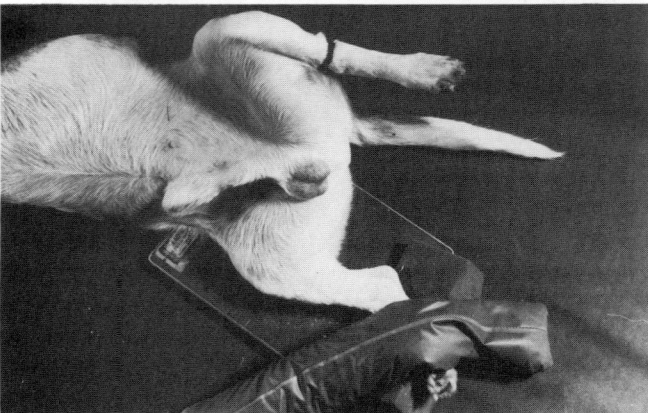

Fig. 41

Postero-anterior hindleg (Fig. 42)

The dog is in sternal recumbency and a sandbag placed under the unaffected limb, so that the body is rotated to the affected side. The affected leg is extended and held in the required position by foam pads and sandbags.

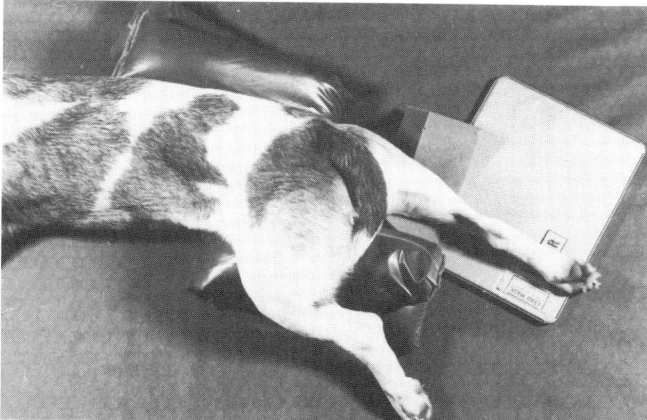

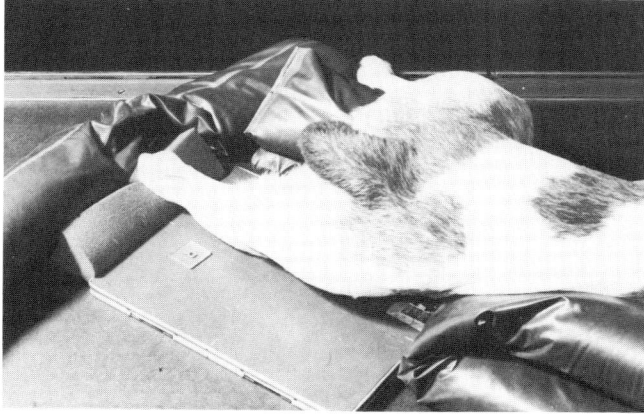

Fig. 42.

Section 2
The Surgical Techniques

Chapter 1
The Repair of the Skin
Techniques for Plastic and Reconstructive Surgery

STEVEN SWAIM

Wound management

Wound debridement, cleansing and bandaging

The protocol for wound debridement will vary depending on the type of wound, the traumatic agent and the environment. For example, the debridement technique for a clean glass cut will be different from that of a crushing–degloving injury incurred in a bacteria-laden environment. Regardless of the technique used, two basic principles apply to any wound debridement technique: (a) removal of contaminated devitalized tissue and foreign debris and (b) thorough lavage of the wound.

Layered debridement is the most common form of debridement and involves removing devitalized tissues beginning at the wound surface and progressing to the depth of the wound. Such debridement is indicated when a wound contains specialized tissues like nerves and tendons. Wounds on the limbs and feet should be debrided in this fashion (Fig. 1.1).

Badly damaged skin edges lacking capillary bleeding should be excised, while keeping in mind that skin may be precious and essential for wound closure. Badly contused or undermined skin edges or evidence of fire or chemical damage to skin will require excision of the affected skin. If doubt exists about skin viability, it may be reinspected 48 h later and excised if necessary. If a skin flap has a sharp line of demarcation between normal and pathologic tissue, the discoloured skin is in danger of sloughing. A skin flap that is slightly discoloured on one end with no sharp demarcation line between normal and abnormal skin will probably survive.

Muscle that appears mushy or friable, does not bleed when cut, does not contract when mechanically stimulated, has dirt ground into it, or is darker or paler than surrounding muscle may be considered non-viable. It has been stated that colour is of questionable value in evaluating muscle viability; however, muscle can be considered viable if it contracts after being stimulated. It is better to remove muscle of doubtful viability than to have it undergo liquifaction necrosis and possible clostridial infection.

When there is an abundance of tissue surrounding a wound, *en bloc* debridement may be used as an effective way of complete wound excision. The wound is packed with sterile gauze, the skin edges are sutured over the gauze, and the entire wound is treated as a tumour. The gauze-packed wound is excised with a margin of normal tissue so that the gauze in the wound is never exposed (Fig. 1.2).

Before, during and after the debriding procedure it is important to *thoroughly* irrigate a wound with *copious* quantities of solution to help eliminate debris and devitalized tissue from the wound as well as remove or dilute bacteria in the wound. A wound lavage solution cleans a wound mechanically by washing away bacteria and debris. A solution may also clean a wound by chemotherapeutics if an antibacterial solution is used. Mechanical cleansing is enhanced by delivering the solution to the wound under moderate pressure using either a 35 ml syringe and 18 gauge needle or a machine[1] that delivers the solution under pulsating or constant pressure.

Sterile isotonic saline and lactated Ringer's solution are both good wound irrigants. However, adding antibacterial agents to a wound lavage solution may increase its cleansing properties. The use of antibacterial agents in wound lavage requires some discretion since any antiseptic strong enough to kill bacteria is strong enough to kill tissue cells. It has been stated that '. . . a biologically oriented surgeon would never select a solution to irrigate a wound which he would not be willing, for instance, to instill into his own conjunctival sac' (Peacock 1984).

Many antibacterial solutions have been used to irrigate wounds. The author prefers a dilute solution of chlorhexidine[2] to irrigate wounds. One part of a 2% concentrate to forty parts of sterile water has been found effective in controlling wound infection.

Following debridement and *thorough* lavage, a wound may be closed by primary wound closure if there is sufficient tissue to allow wound closure and if the surgeon is convinced that healing will progress without interruption by wound infection. Suture materials to close the deep tissues in such wounds include chromic catgut, undyed polyglycolic acid suture,[3] undyed polygalactin 910,[4] monofilament polypropylene[5] and nylon.[6] The latter two plus polymerized caprolactum[7] and stainless steel can be used for skin closure.

If *any* doubt exists in the surgeon's mind as to any remaining wound contamination, a drain should be placed in the wound prior to closure and left in place until drainage subsides and there are no signs of wound infection. Antimicrobial solutions may be flushed through such drains. The wound should be bandaged with a non-adherent absorbent pad[8] followed by a secondary dressing and tape to hold the pad in place. The dressing should be changed daily.

If a wound is undoubtedly contaminated or infected, it should be left open and be properly dressed. Once infection is controlled, the wound can be: (a) closed by delayed primary closure (i.e. within 3–5 days after infliction); (b) allowed to form granulation tissue and be closed by secondary closure (i.e. after 5 days from infliction); or (c) be allowed to heal by second intention.

When dressing infected wounds, topical medications such as enzymatic debriding agents and/or antibiotics may be applied to the wound or the covering to be placed on the

---

[1] Water-Pik®, Teledyne Aquatic Corp., Ft. Collins, CO 80521.
[2] Nolvosan®, Ft Dodge Laboratories, Inc., Ft Dodge, Iowa 50501.
[3] Dexon, Davis and Geck (Lederle-Cyanamid), Pearl River, NY 10965.
[4] Vicryl, Ethicon, Inc., Somerville, NJ 08876.

[5] Prolene, Ethicon, Inc., Somerville, NJ 08876.
[6] Ethilon, Ethicon, Inc., Somerville, NJ 08876.
[7] Supramid, S. Jackson, Inc., Washington, DC.
[8] Telfa-Wet Pruf Pad, The Kendall Co., Boston, MA.

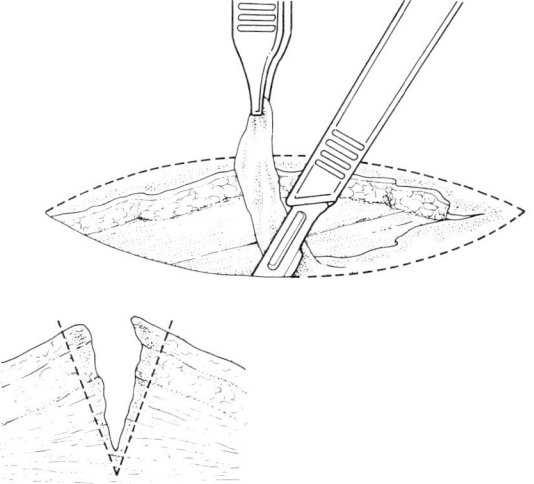

Fig. 1.1. Layered wound debridement begins at the surface of the wound and progresses to the depths of the wound (redrawn from Archibald, 1974).

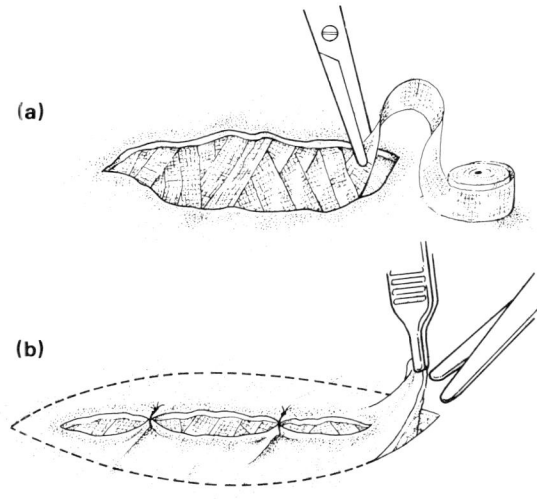

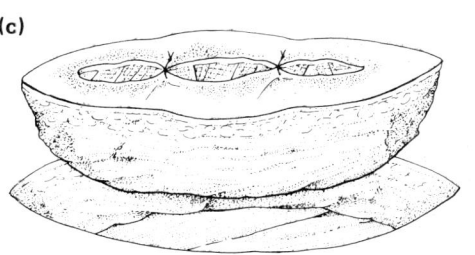

Fig. 1.2. *En bloc* wound debridement. The wound is packed with surgical gauze (a); the wound edges are temporarily sutured, and the wound is excised using the technique of tumour excision with a margin of normal tissue being removed with the wound (b and c) (redrawn from Swaim, 1980).

wound. Initial wound dressing materials should be absorbent, thus allowing the absorption of exudate and tissue debris into the bandage in the early phases of wound healing. Sterile saline saturated surgical sponges, with or without antibiotic solution in them, may be applied to wounds followed by a dry absorbent bandage material[9] and a tertiary dressing material[10] and tape to hold the bandage in place. The dressings should be changed once or twice daily to remove absorbed debris and exudate from the wound.

As granulation tissue forms in the wound, a non-adherent absorbent dressing material should be placed over the wound followed by a teriary dressing and tape to hold the bandage in place. The need for bandage changes is usually less frequent once granulation tissue has formed in the wound.

Shifting local tissue to close defects

The simplest means of closing skin defects is shifting local tissues around the wound to close it. Because of the loose elastic skin of the dog and cat, many skin defects may be closed in this manner. Wounds may be closed by various techniques depending upon the shape of the wound. The following are some of the more common wound closure techniques. For more information on the subject, the reader is referred to other sources.

Fusiform-shaped wounds are the most common shaped defect. They are easily closed by layered closure, resulting

[9] Wet Pruf Pad, The Kendall Co., Boston, MA.
[10] Kerlix roll, The Kendall Co., Boston, MA.

in a straight linear scar. The length to width ratio of such a defect should approach 4:1 to help avoid 'dog-ears' that might form at the ends of the suture line during closure (Fig. 1.3a).

When skin is available on all sides of a triangular, square or rectangular defect, suturing should progress from the corners towards the centre of the defect. Sutures are placed alternately at the corners of the defect until the defect is closed. The result is a Y-, X-, or double Y-shaped scar respectively (Fig. 1.3b–d).

Closing crescent-shaped defects entails suturing two skin edges of unequal length together. One technique to accomplish this is the placement of a central suture in the defect followed by suturing from this point to the ends of the defect. The 'dog-ears' that form at the ends of the suture line are then removed (Fig. 1.3e).

Chevron-shaped defects also have one side of the defect longer than the other side because of the small flap of skin associated with the defect. Closure begins at the base of the defect and progresses until tension begins to develop on the sutures. At this point the remaining sides of the lesion are sutured to the edges of the flap to produce a Y-shaped scar (Fig. 1.3f).

Circular defects can be converted to fusiform defects and closed as previously described (Fig. 1.3g). Another technique to close circular defects in thin skin is to pull three or four points equidistant around the defect into the centre of the defect using a single suture. The remaining side arms of the defect are closed and 'dog-ears' are removed to produce either a Y-shaped (if three points are used) or X-shaped (if four points are used) scar (Fig. 1.3h).

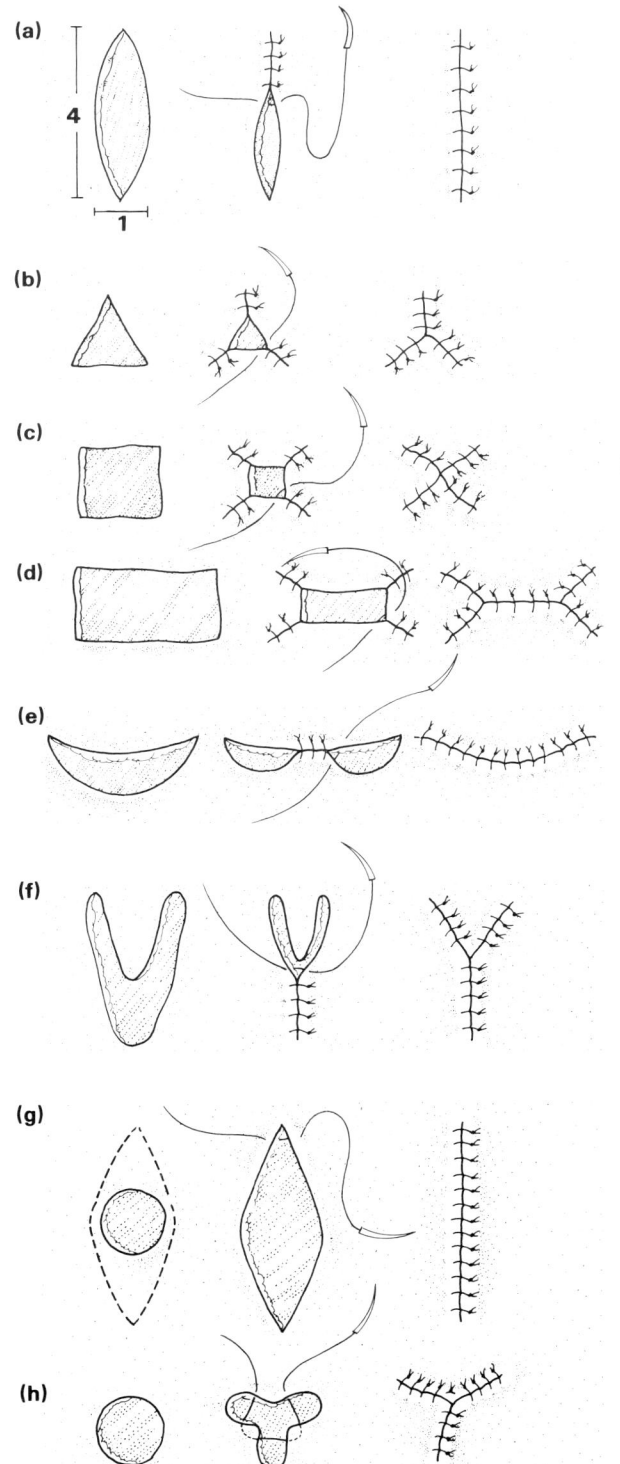

Fig. 1.3. Techniques for closing various shaped wounds. (a) Fusiform: should have a 4 : 1 length to width ratio; (b) triangle; (c) square; (d) rectangle: centripetal closure from the corners; (e) crescent: centrifugal closure from the wound's centre with 'dog-ear' removal as necessary; (f) chevron: closure of wound's base followed by closure of the side arms; (g) circle: conversion to a fusiform wound followed by closure; (h) circle: conversion to a 3-armed wound followed by closure of the arms with 'dog-ear' removal as necessary.

Selected practical techniques for wound repair

'Walking' sutures

'Walking' sutures are used in both small and large wounds on dogs. They can be used in areas where skin is abundant and where skin is sparse. Walking sutures are especially useful on the trunk and other areas of the body where the skin is loosely attached and readily moved. These sutures provide a means of: (a) moving skin from around a wound to cover the wound, (b) obliterating dead space, and (c) evenly distributing tension to the tissues around the wound rather than concentrating tension at the wound's edge as do other tension sutures. Moving surrounding skin to cover the defect is advantageous because it reduces the time and care needed for treating wounds by skin grafts or by allowing them to heal by wound contraction. Obliteration of dead space helps to reduce the possibility of haematoma formation. The even distribution of tension around a wound rather than the concentration of tension at the wound edge helps prevent wound disruption.

The skin around the wound is undermined; care is taken to leave intact any large blood vessels coming from underlying tissues to the dermis. Using 2-0 or 3-0 absorbable suture material with a swaged needle, the first walking suture is placed near the junction of the under-mined skin with the underlying tissue. The first portion of the suture is placed by passing the needle through the deep portion of the dermis but not through the full thickness of the skin. By observing the deep portion of the dermis, the incorporation of large blood vessels into the suture can be avoided, thereby assuring adequate blood supply to the skin. The second bite of the suture is taken in the underlying tissue toward the centre of the wound. As the suture is tied, skin is advanced slightly toward the centre of the wound because of its elasticity (Figs 1.4 and 1.5).*

Walking sutures are placed in rows, thereby moving skin across the defect. After two or three rows of sutures have been placed, the skin is usually half-way across the wound. Repeating the same procedure on the opposite side of the wound results in almost complete closure of the wound. When a wound is adjacent to another body structure or orifice (e.g. eye or anus), walking sutures advance skin from only one side of the wound to prevent distortion of the structure or orifice.

A simple continuous subcuticular suture of 2-0 or 3-0 absorbable suture material is placed along the wound edge to approximate the tissues. Final closure of the skin is accomplished with simple interrupted non-absorbable sutures that are placed close to the skin's edges. There is no tension on these final sutures (Fig. 1.6).

* Figs 1.5, 1.15–1.22 are based on photographs from Swaim S.F. (1980) *Surgery of Traumatized Skin: Management and Reconstruction in the Dog and Cat.* W.B. Saunders Co., Philadelphia.

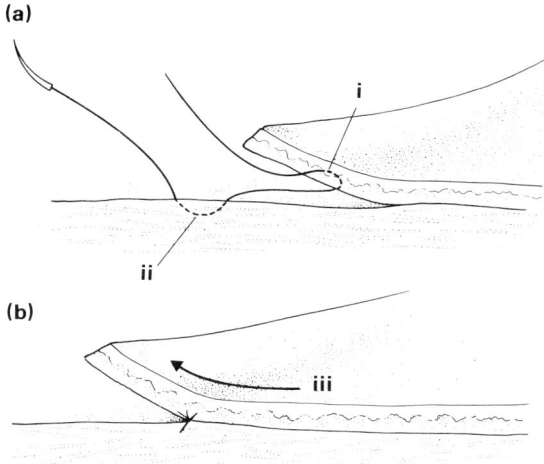

(a)

i

ii

(b)

iii

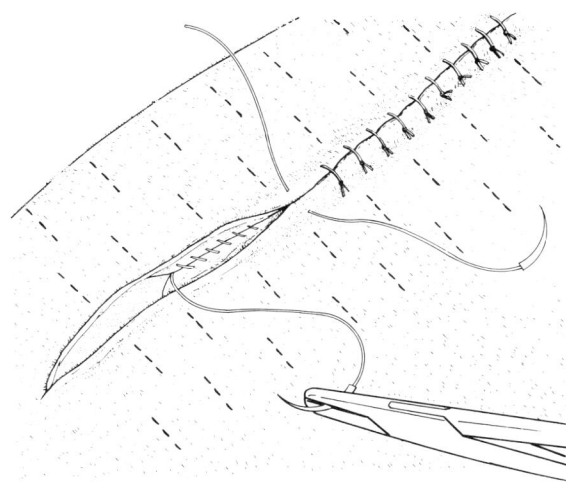

Fig. 1.4 (a) Placement of a 'walking' suture with 2-0 or 3-0 absorbable suture material. The first suture bite (i) is in the deep dermis and the second bite (ii) is in the underlying tissue toward the wound's centre. (b) Tying the suture moves the skin slightly toward the wound's centre (iii). (From Swaim, 1980.)

Fig. 1.6. Final closure of a wound in which 'walking' sutures have been used. Subcuticular 'walking' sutures (broken lines), simple continuous subcuticular suture, simple interrupted skin sutures.

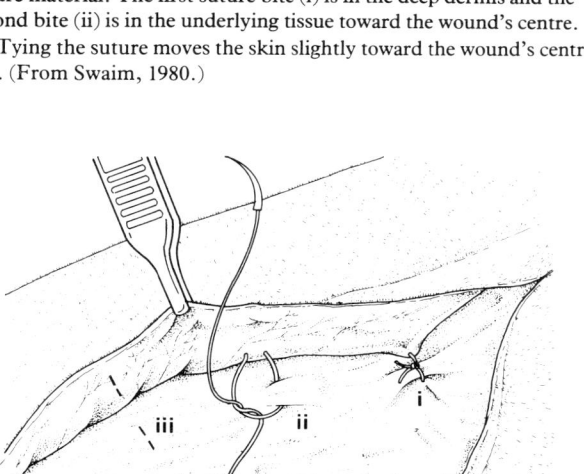

Fig. 1.5. Placement and tying of a row of 'walking' sutures. Tying the first suture advances the skin toward the wound's centre (i). The second suture of the row has been placed (ii). Points of insertion of the third suture (iii).

Rotation flaps

A rotation flap is a semicircular or three-fourths circular flap of skin and subcutaneous tissue that rotates about a pivot point to close a skin defect. Triangular skin defects lend themselves to this type of closure. Rotation flaps are useful for closing defects where skin is only available on one side of the defect (e.g. lesions around the eye or anus). The technique is also useful in areas where obtaining skin from one side of the lesion would result in distortion of structures covered by that skin (e.g. prepuce or scrotum) (Fig. 1.7). The technique can also be used bilaterally to close large triangular defects and/or triangular defects where skin for reconstruction is only available on two sides of the defect (Fig. 1.8).

As a flap is rotated and sutured into its new position, redundant skin begins to appear along the outer side of the suture line as suturing progresses, thus forming a 'dog ear' of skin at the end of the suture line. This is removed as a triangle of skin after it develops or as a triangle of skin (Bürow's triangle) before closure begins (Fig. 1.9).

Flaps that rotate have a tendency to shorten and develop a diagonal line of tension across the flap as they move into their new position. Therefore, rotation flaps should be designed to prevent such tension. The larger the radius of the flap, the less is the tension, and it rotates into position easier (Fig. 1.10a). The rule of having the incision from a rotation flap four times longer than the distance through which the flap will rotate may not be as critical in the dog and cat as it is in man because of the elasticity of dog and cat skin. However, flaps should be made large enough to avoid tension on surrounding tissues, especially when the tension may result in distortion of nearby tissues (e.g. ectropion).

Tension across a rotation flap may also be prevented by making a back cut into the base of the flap to relax the tension and allow the flap to move by a combination of rotation and transposition. The back cut should be made carefully so that it does not extend too far into the base of the flap, thereby interfering with the flap's blood supply. The back cut can be made selectively through only the skin leaving the blood supply in the subcutaneous tissue intact to supply the flap (Fig. 1.10b).

Tension on a flap may also be avoided by extending the length of the side of the flap adjacent to the defect (Fig. 1.10c). A small stab incision made in the centre of the line of tension and perpendicular to it is another way to help relieve tension across a rotation flap (Fig. 1.10d).

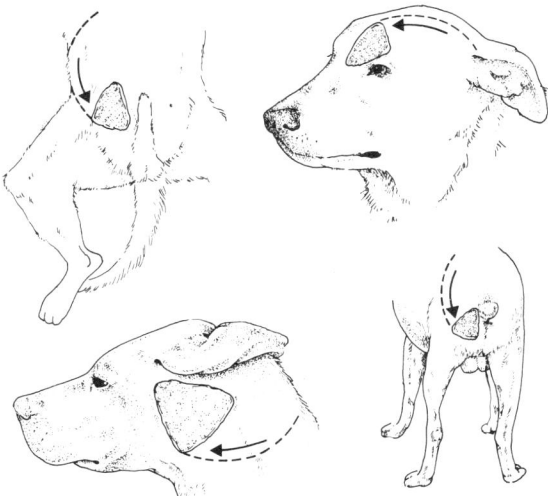

Fig. 1.7. Areas where rotation flaps would be indicated—where skin is available on only one side of the defect (e.g. eyes, ears, or anus); where moving skin from one side of the defect would result in distortion of structures in the area (e.g. prepuce) (redrawn from Swaim, 1978).

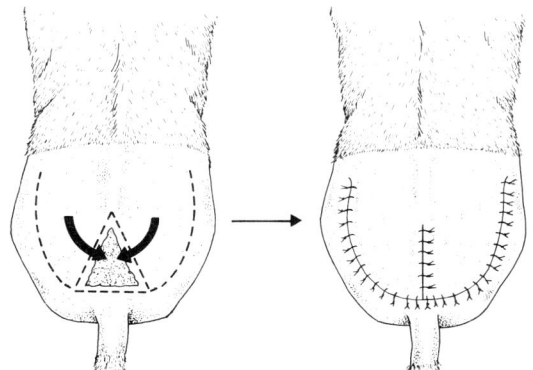

Fig. 1.8. Bilateral rotation flaps used to close a triangular shaped skin defect over a dog's lumbosacral area (redrawn from Swaim, 1982).

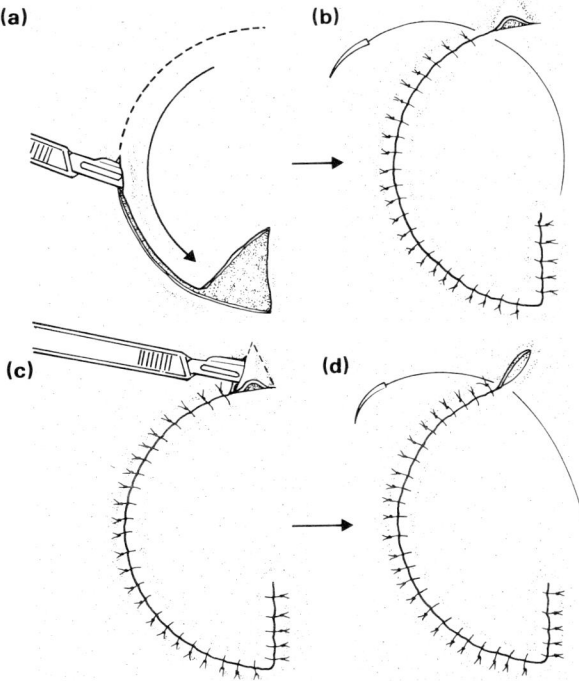

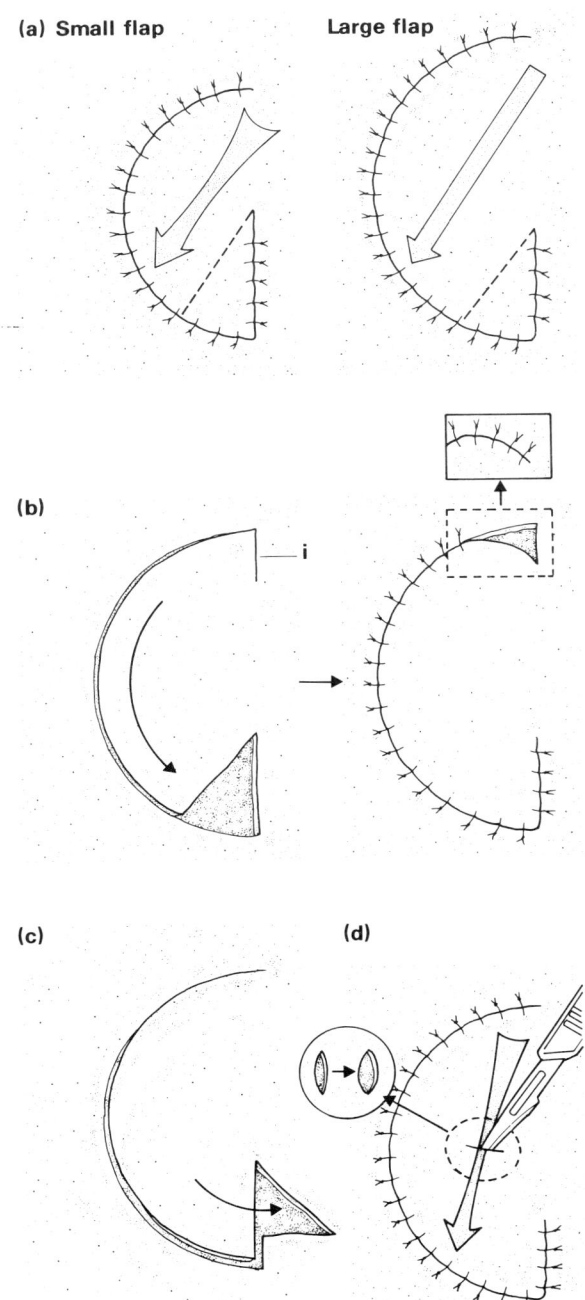

Fig. 1.10. Techniques to prevent tension on rotation flaps. (a) Design large flaps as smaller flaps increase tension; (b) make a back cut into the flap's base (i); (c) slight extension of the side of the flap adjacent to the lesion; (d) make a stab incision perpendicular to the line of tension. (From Archibald, in press.)

Fig. 1.9. Dynamics of a rotation flap. (a) Incision and rotation of a semi-circular skin flap. (b) Suturing flap in place with 'dog-ear' formation. (c) Removal of the 'dog-ear'. (d) Final closure of area where 'dog-ear' was removed.

Single pedicle advancement flaps

A single pedicle advancement flap is a mobilized skin flap that is moved into a defect without changing the plane of the pedicle. These flaps can be used to correct defects around which the skin is loose and abundant. The skin's elasticity is used to advance the flap to cover the wound. As with rotation flaps, these flaps can be used to correct defects which have skin available on only one side of the defect and defects with skin available on two sides (Fig. 1.11).

Single pedicle advancement flaps are basically rectangular in shape. Triangles of skin (Bürow's triangles) can be excised lateral to the base of the flap. This helps equalize the length of the sides of the flap and the adjacent wound margins. The base of these triangles should be as long as the lesion to be covered (Fig. 1.12).

To help alleviate some of the tension on a flap, back-cuts can be made into the flap's base. These back-cuts open into 'V's' as the flap is advanced over the defect. Tension on the flap is relieved as the 'V's' approach a straight line (Fig. 1.13a). Back-cuts should not be made too far into the flap's base, otherwise its blood supply could be damaged. This problem can be circumvented by cutting the flap's base wider so the pedicle remains wide enough to furnish a good blood supply to the flap (Fig. 1.13a). Another technique that can be used to help elongate a flap is to angulate or curve the sides of the flap away from each other (Fig. 1.13b and 1.13c). Modified Z-plasties can also be used at the base of the flap as a means of helping elongate the flap (Fig. 1.13d). Walking sutures can be used to advance a flap into position, thereby gradually elongating the flap and distributing tension along the flap.

When two apposing single pedicle advancement flaps are used to reconstruct a square or rectangular defect, the result is an H-plasty. Each flap of the H-plasty should be at least as long as half the width of the defect to be covered. However, each flap may be made as long as the defect is wide, particularly if tension will be great. If Bürow's triangles are removed adjacent to the base of each flap, the length of the base of each triangle should be half the width of the defect to be closed (Fig. 1.14). Vertical mattress tension sutures can be used to help appose the edges of the two flaps, and simple interrupted sutures are used for final skin closure. As an alternative, walking sutures can be used as tension sutures to advance the flaps together.

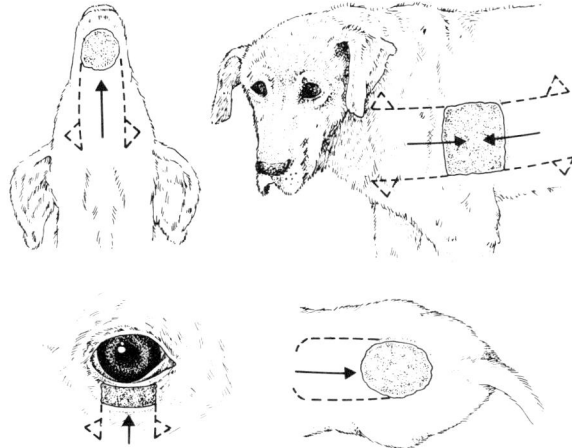

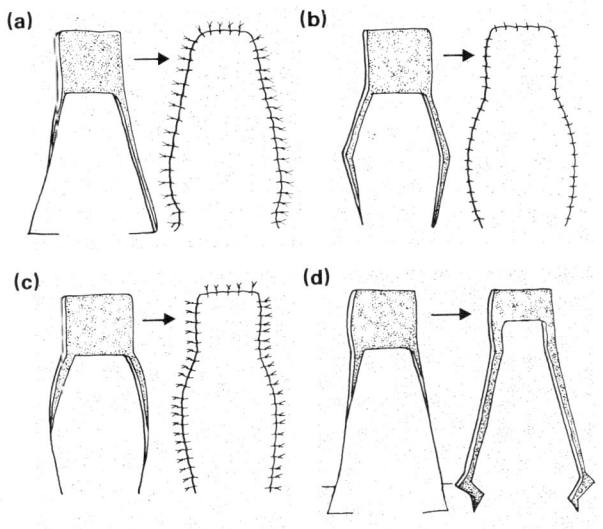

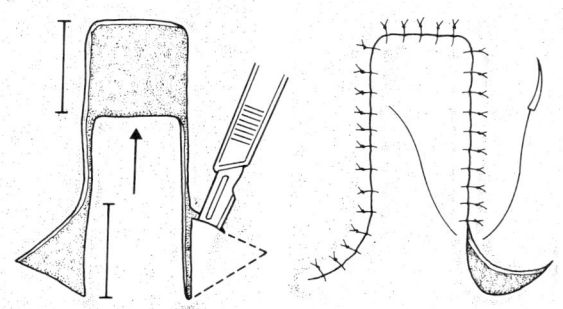

Fig. 1.11. Areas where single pedicle advancement flaps would be indicated — where skin is loose and abundant on one or both sides of a defect (redrawn from Swaim, 1978).

Fig. 1.12. Single pedicle advancement flap with Bürow's triangles being removed lateral to the base of the flap to help equalize the length of the sides of the flap and adjacent wound margins. The base of each triangle and the width of the defect are equal.

Fig. 1.13. Techniques to help present tension on single pedicle advancement flaps. (a) Widened base with back cuts; (b) widened flap centre (angulated); (c) widened flap centre (curved); (d) modified Z-plasty at flap base. (b, c and d redrawn from Converse, 1977.)

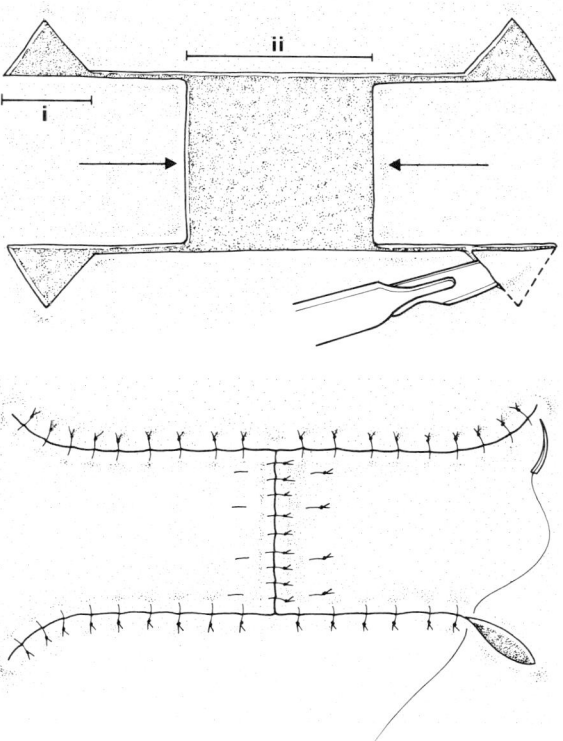

Fig. 1.14. Two single pedicle advancement flaps (H-plasty) used to close a square defect. The length of the flaps and length of the defect are equal. The bases of Bürow's triangles are ½ (i) the width of the defect (ii). If needed, vertical mattress sutures can be used at the junction of the flaps to help relieve tension (redrawn from Archibald, in press).

Pouch flaps (distant double pedicle direct flap)

A pouch flap is a double pedicle flap that is created on the body and used to reconstruct a defect on an extremity by moving the extremity to the flap. These flaps provide an economical, cosmetic, and functional form of skin reconstruction on the limbs. Such flaps are economical because they are constructed and placed on the limb in one stage and separated from the body in a second stage. They are cosmetic since they provide a full-thickness, fully haired piece of skin for reconstruction. Pouch flaps are functional because such skin will withstand the trauma it will be subjected to on the distal limb. These flaps have the advantage of having two pedicles (i.e. one dorsal and one ventral) which help hold the flap against the body while vascular linkage develops between the flap and the defect.

The size and temperament of an animal should be considered before using a pouch flap. A small dog or cat could more readily have a limb bandaged along their side than a giant breed of dog. Additionally, some animals may not tolerate having their limb bandaged along their side, regardless of their size.

The lateral thoraco-abdominal area and the limb to be reconstructed, including the foot on that limb, should be thoroughly prepared for aseptic surgery. The animal is placed in lateral recumbency with the affected limb uppermost. The superficial tissue (i.e. granulation tissue and epithelialized granulation tissue) on the wound is shaved off at a depth of about 1–2 mm to include removal of a narrow margin of normal tissue at the wound's edge. The defect is covered with a saline moistened surgical sponge while the flap is prepared.

Two parallel dorso–ventral incisions are made on the lateral aspect of the thorax or abdomen. The distance between the incisions is equal to the dorso–ventral dimension of the limb defect (Fig. 1.15). The flap is undermined, the limb is flexed, and the foot is passed under the flap. The limb is moved until the defect lies under the flap. Simple interrupted sutures are used to suture the edges of the flap and wound together. The flap is sutured around the limb as far as possible in an attempt to 'wrap' the flap around the limb (Fig. 1.16). Two or three tacking sutures may be placed to immobilize the flap to the defect. A small Penrose drain should be placed in the most dependent base of the flap to allow for drainage of any fluid that may accumulate in the space around the limb and flap (Fig. 1.17).

Periodic bandage changes, systemic antibiotics, topical antibiotics, and antibiotic flushes of the limb–flap area may be used to control any infection that might develop. Any flushing under the limb–flap area should be performed carefully with a non-caustic solution to prevent mechanical and chemical damage to the vascular linkages occurring between the flap and defect.

The limb is immobilized against the body for approximately 14 days, with periodic bandage changes especially if there is copious drainage. After approximately 14 days, the attachments of the flap to the side of the animal are cut free, trimmed and sutured to the remaining wound margins of the defect. Adequate skin should be taken from the thoraco–abdominal area when cutting the bases of the flap free. This assures sufficient skin to complete closure of the limb lesion (Fig. 1.18). The skin's mobility over the thoraco–abdominal area permits the surgeon to close the donor site by undermining and advancing the skin edges together with walking sutures or tension sutures and skin apposition sutures (Fig. 1.19).

If the development of adequate blood supply in the flap is questionable after 14 days, the flap may be left attached to the body longer, or it may be separated from the body in stages as a surgical delaying technique (i.e. severing one pedicle of the flap followed by severance of the second pedicle 3–5 days later).

After a flap has been completely transferred to the limb, it should be protected by a bandage for another 10 days.

The single pedicle direct flap is a modification of the pouch flap. The technique for constructing this type of flap is basically the same as for a pouch flap. The difference is that this flap has only one pedicle as opposed to two on the pouch flap, thus there is more dependance on adequate bandaging to hold the limb against the body.

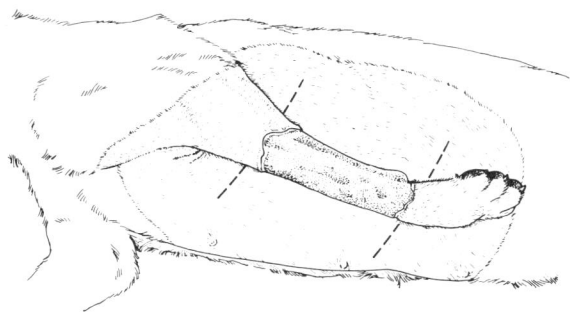

Fig. 1.15. Degloving injury on the forelimb of a dog. Limb is positioned along the thoracic area. Broken lines indicate incisions to create ends of a pouch flap.

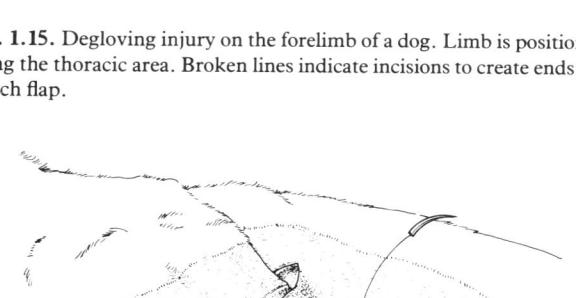

Fig. 1.16. The limb has been placed through the pouch flap. The edges of the flap are being sutured to the edges of the lesion.

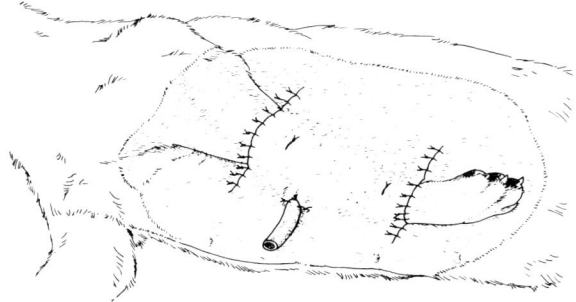

Fig. 1.17. The pouch flap has been sutured around the limb as far as possible. Tacking sutures have been placed to anchor the flap to the lesion. A Penrose drain has been placed under the dependent area of the flap to allow drainage of tissue fluids.

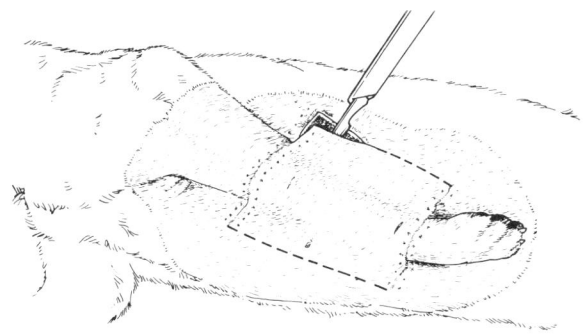

Fig. 1.18. After 2 weeks, the pedicles of the pouch flap are incised from the thoracic area. Adequate tissue is taken with the pedicles of the flap to allow for closure of the remaining defect on the medial aspect of the limb.

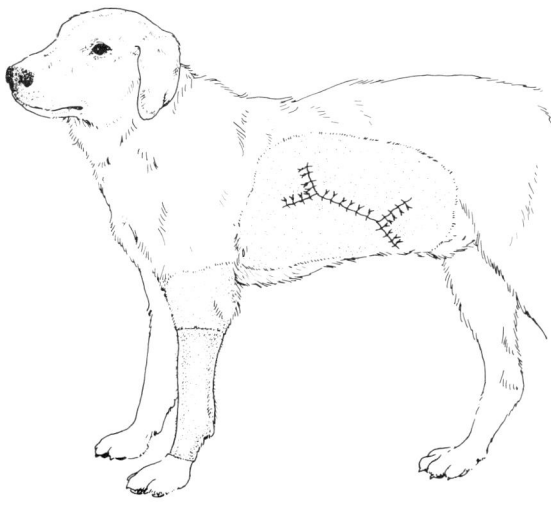

Fig. 1.19. Completed transfer of pouch flap to the forelimb with centripetal closure of the rectangular defect left at the thoracic donor site.

Mesh grafts

A practical skin graft is a mesh graft made from a full-thickness piece of skin in which numerous slits have been cut in parallel rows. The indications for a mesh graft are related to the three advantages of these grafts. First, the slits in the graft allow the graft to expand so a large wound can be covered by a piece of skin that is smaller than the wound. Second, these grafts can be applied to less than ideal graft beds (e.g. ones where exudate, blood and serum are present). The slits in the graft allow drainage from the wound. Third, mesh grafts can be used to cover irregular (undulating) surfaces that are difficult to immobilize. The slits allow the graft to conform to the wound surface better, and tacking sutures can be placed between the slits to immobilize the graft on its bed. A fourth advantage of mesh grafts is that a large percentage (95–100%) of each graft takes.

The disadvantages of a mesh graft are that: (a) they have an uncosmetic appearance initially because of the slits, (b) they may take longer to heal, and (c) the adnexa of the skin are more widely dispersed. These disadvantages are encountered when large slits are cut in a graft and the graft is expanded to its maximum to cover the wound.

A piece of sterile towelling is laid over the wound to obtain a pattern of the wound. This pattern is cut out and placed on the graft donor site, the lateral thoracic area that has been prepared for aseptic surgery. The pattern is placed so that the direction of hair growth on the graft will be the same as the direction of hair growth on the skin around the wound. After tracing around the pattern with sterile methylene blue on a sterile tooth pick, the full thickness of the skin is incised along the tracing line. The graft is elevated from the donor site (Fig. 1.20).

The donor site can be closed by undermining and advancing the skin edges together with walking sutures or tension sutures and skin apposition sutures. To save time, an assistant surgeon can do this while the surgeon prepares the graft for application to the defect.

The graft is placed dermal side up on a piece of sterile cardboard in which slits have been cut around the edges. Pieces of 2-0 silk are placed through the graft's edges at sufficient points around the graft so that it can be stretched out evenly on the cardboard. The silk sutures are drawn through the slits at the edges of the cardboard to stretch the graft out.

A pair of Metzenbaum scissors and thumb forceps are used to remove all remaining subcutaneous tissue from the graft so that it contains only dermis and epidermis (Fig. 1.21). A No. 11 scalpel blade is then used to cut staggered parallel rows of slits in the graft. The slits are about 1.0–1.5 cm long and 2.5–5.0 mm apart (Fig. 1.22).

The graft is removed from the cardboard, the silk sutures are removed from the skin edge and the graft is laid on the wound. One edge of the graft is sutured to its corresponding wound edge using simple interrupted sutures of 3-0 to 4-0 non-absorbable suture material (i.e. polypropylene). The graft is stretched slightly so that it overlaps the opposite wound edge by 2–3 mm, and the overlapped skin is excised followed by suturing the remaining graft edge to the wound edge (Fig. 1.23). This slight stretching opens the slits in the graft enough to allow for drainage, and yet does not open the slits so wide as to leave wide open areas that could prolong both the healing time and the time needed to regain a cosmetic appearance. Drainage is a major feature in obtaining the total or near total take of a mesh graft.

The minimally expanded mesh graft described above is primarily indicated for wounds on the limbs where the total skin necessary for wound coverage can be easily obtained from the trunk.

Once the graft has been sutured to the wound edges, simple interrupted tacking sutures can be placed between some mesh holes in the graft to secure it to the bed. Such sutures should especially be placed at points where the graft does not readily contact the graft bed.

After sutured in place, a non-adherent wound dressing-pad[11] is placed over the graft, and this is covered with a soft absorbent wound wrapping material. Adhesive tape covers this wrapping, and a splint may be incorporated in the bandage to assure wound immobilization. The bandage should be changed daily to remove any drainage from the grafted area. As drainage becomes less, bandage changes can be done less frequently. In the presence of infection, a thin coating of antibiotic ointment may be placed on the non-adherent dressing pad. Twenty-one days after grafting the graft should be sufficiently healed in place and durable enough to discontinue bandages.

As the graft takes and matures, the mesh holes heal and wound contraction makes them less obvious. As hair grows back on the graft, it becomes even more cosmetic (Fig. 1.24). If the holes are expanded minimally, the graft becomes more cosmetic sooner.

[11] Telfa-Pad, The Kendall Co., Boston, Ma.

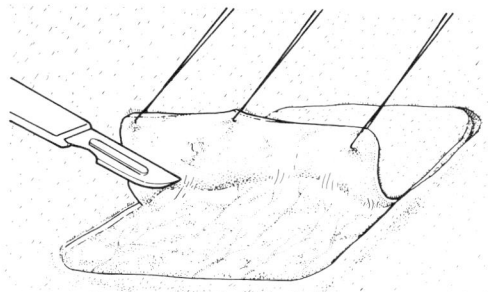

Fig. 1.20. A full-thickness skin graft being elevated by stay sutures while a scalpel blade is used to remove the graft from the donor site (lateral thoracic area).

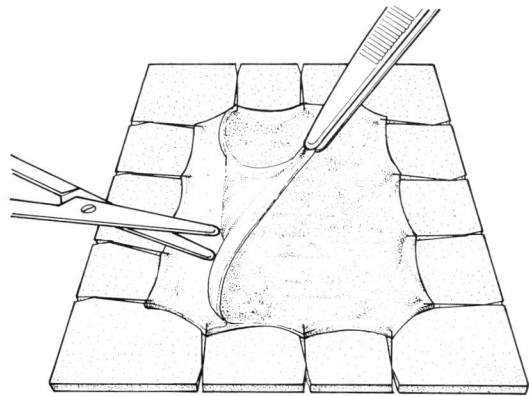

Fig. 1. 21. The skin graft has been fixed, dermal side up, to a piece of sterile cardboard by means of silk sutures pulled through slits in the edge of the cardboard. Blunt pointed scissors and dressing forceps are being used to remove all remaining subcutaneous tissue from the dermis.

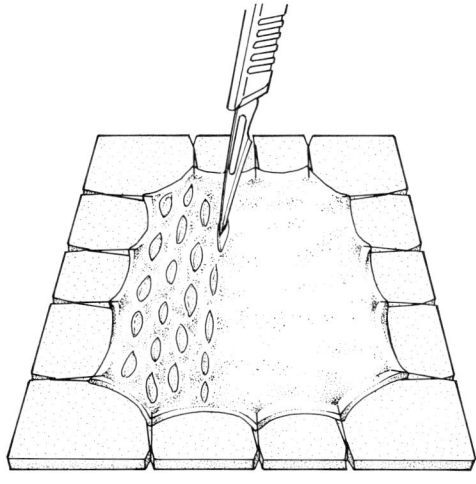

Fig. 1.22. A No. 11 scalpel blade being used to cut staggered parallel rows of slits in the graft. Slits are 1.0–1.5 cm long and about 2.5–5.0 mm apart.

(a)

(b)

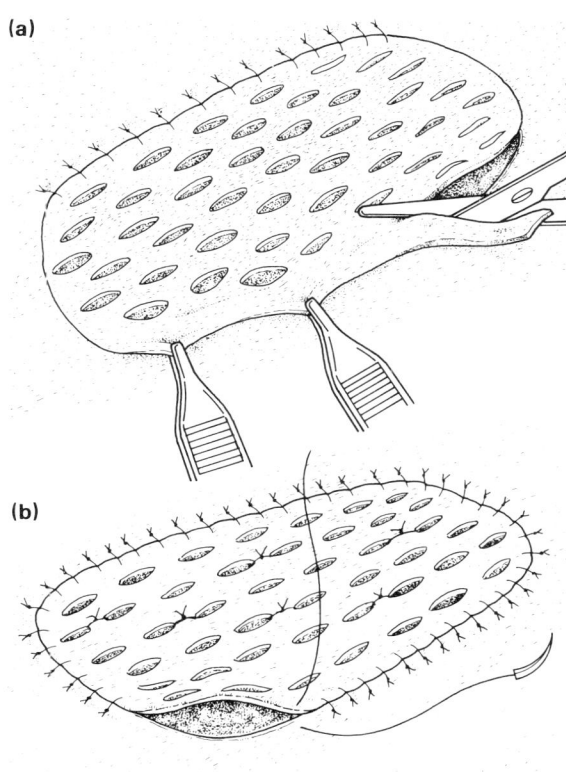

Fig. 1.23. The mesh graft has been sutured to one edge of the wound and stretched slightly to overlap the opposite wound edge by 2–3 mm. (a) The overlapped skin is removed. (b) The remaining edge of the graft is sutured to the remaining wound edge and tacking sutures are placed through some of the mesh holes to anchor the graft to its bed.

Fig. 1.24. Healed mesh graft. As mesh holes heal by epithelialization and contraction, they become smaller and less noticeable. As hair regrows on the graft it becomes even more cosmetic.

Strip grafts

Strip grafts are strips of full-thickness skin 3–4 mm wide that are placed in parallel linear grooves that have been cut in a bed of granulation tissue. These grafts are primarily indicated to reconstruct skin defects on the limbs of animals. Because of their narrowness, their placement in granulation tissue and wound drainage they allow, strip grafts usually take well. The granulation tissue between the strips is covered by epithelium that spreads from the edges of the strip grafts as they heal in place. Initially, the grafted area has an uncosmetic appearance because of these epithelialized areas. As the grafts mature, they become wider, the epithelialized areas between grafts become narrower and the grafts grow hair, all of which help to make the grafted area appear more cosmetic.

After a bed of healthy granulation tissue has formed on the wound, a No. 15 scalpel blade is used to cut parallel grooves in the granulation tissue. These grooves are cut about 2–3 mm deep and about 3 mm wide (Fig. 1.25). When cut at this width, the groove will tend to widen after the strip of granulation tissue is removed. After all of the grooves have been cut the wound is covered with a gauze soaked in sterile physiologic saline.

A sterile toothpick dipped in sterile methylene blue can be used to draw strips on the lateral thoracic donor area which has been prepared for aspetic surgery. These strips of skin should be drawn slightly wider (4–5 mm) than the final width of the grooves in the granulation tissue. This will allow for the primary contraction of the strip when it is removed from the body.

Each strip is incised with a scalpel and removed as a full-thickness piece of skin (Fig. 1.26). Any subcutaneous fat or tissue adhering to the dermis of the strip should be removed. The strip is laid into one of the previously prepared grooves, being certain that the direction of hair growth on the graft is like that of the area surrounding the graft.

A simple interrupted non-absorbable suture is used to tack each end of the graft to the skin at the end of the groove. If necessary, other sutures may be used to immobilize the strip graft to the sides of the groove in selected areas to help immobilize the graft in its groove (Fig. 1.27).

Postoperative bandaging of strip grafts is the same as for mesh grafts. As the grafts take, epithelial tissue grows from the edges of each strip to cover the granulation tissue between strips. The grafts become wider as they mature and some hair regrows on the grafts. The grafted area is not as cosmetic as the surrounding area, but it has wound coverage (Fig. 1.28).

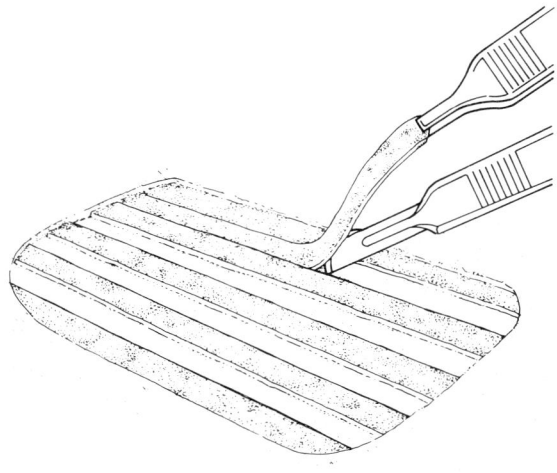

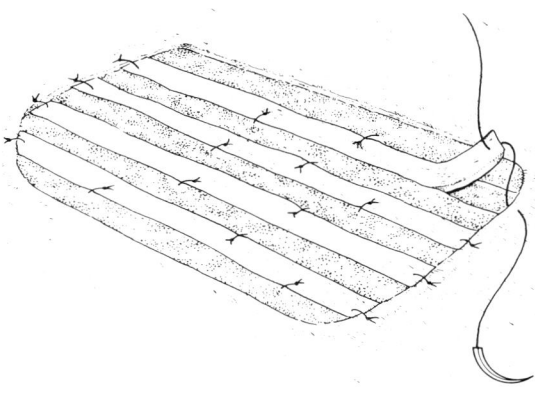

Fig. 1.25. A No. 15 scalpel blade is used to cut parallel grooves in the granulation tissue. Grooves are cut about 2–3 mm deep and 3 mm wide. As tissue is removed from the groove, the groove widens slightly.

Fig. 1.27. Each skin strip is laid in a previously prepared groove and anchored at each end with a simple interrupted suture. Other simple interrupted sutures are placed where needed to immobilize the strip in its groove.

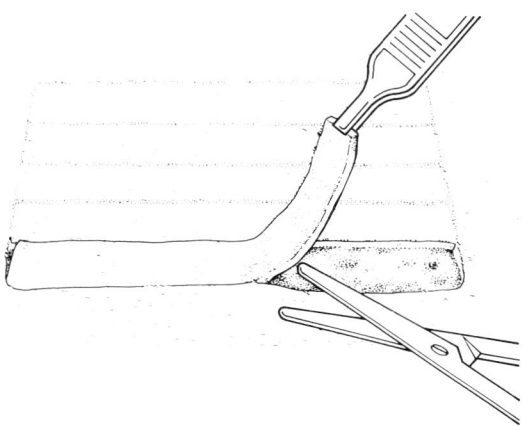

Fig. 1.26. Methylene blue is used to draw strips of skin about 4–5 mm wide on the donor area–lateral thorax. Each strip is incised with a scalpel blade and elevated from the donor area. All subcutaneous tissue is removed from each graft.

Fig. 1.28. As strip grafts take, epithelial tissue grows over exposed granulation tissue from the edges of each graft, the grafts become wider as they mature, and some hair regrows on each graft. The grafted area is not as cosmetic as the surrounding area, but it has wound coverage.

Chapter 2
Surgery of the Head and Neck Region

PETER G. C. BEDFORD

Ablation of the vertical part of the external auditory canal

Indications

Chronic otitis externa in which integumental hyperplasia has led to gross attenuation of the external auditory canal. Lateral wall resection would lead to increased aeration and drainage, but the medial wall of the vertical part of the canal would still prove a source of inflammation and discomfort.

Equipment

A routine surgical set.

Technique

The patient is positioned in lateral recumbency, and the peri-aural skin and pinna clipped and prepared in the usual way. A T-shaped incision is made thrugh the skin to expose the conchal cartilage. The arms of the T extend along the lateral margin of the tragus whilst the upright of the T extends to below the level of the horizontal part of the external auditory canal (Fig. 2.1a). The two skin flaps formed are reflected, and any parotid gland tissue overlying the conchal cartilage is dissected free (Fig. 2.1b and 2.2). Dissection continues around the medial side of the cartilage until the cartilage remains attached only at the level of the tragus dorsally and the horizontal canal ventrally (Figs 2.1c and 2.3). The arms of the original T incision are continued around the edge of the tragus and along the base of the pinna to free the proximal part of the canal completely (Figs 2.1d and 2.4a). The cartilage is then sectioned at the level of the horizontal part of the canal (Fig. 2.1e and 2.4b), and the two skin flaps are sutured to close the wound, leaving the meatus of the horizontal canal open (Figs 2.1f and 2.5).

Postoperative care

Bandaging is not necessary, but self-trauma can be prevented by using an Elizabethan collar. Routine antibiosis.

Possible complications

Cartilage necrosis and wound breakdown can lead to occlusion of the entrance to the meatus.

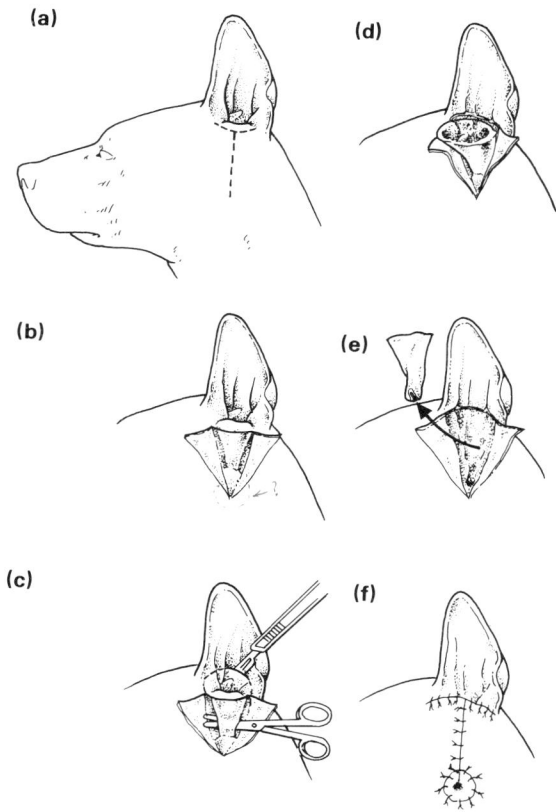

Fig. 2.1. Schematic diagram of the technique to ablate the vertical part of the external auditory canal. (a) The T-shaped skin incision; (b) exposure of the conchal cartilage; (c) dissection of the medial aspect of the conchal cartilage; (d) the conchal cartilage has been freed from the base of the pinna; (e) excision of the vertical part of the external auditory canal; (f) closure.

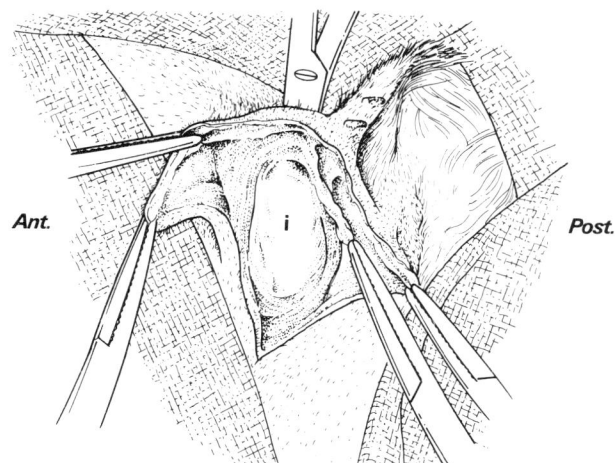

Fig. 2.2. Exposure of the lateral aspect of the conchal cartilage (i).

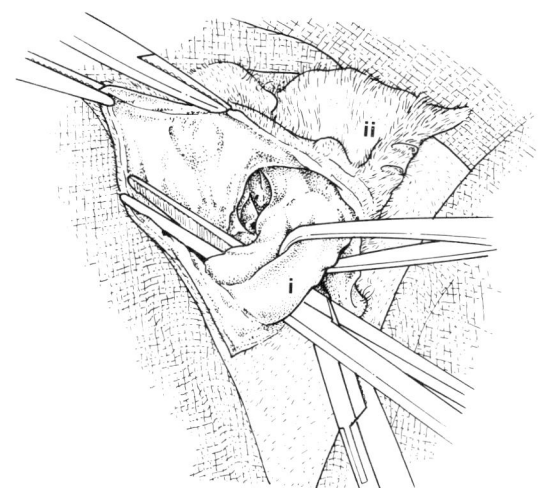

Fig. 2.3. Dissection of the medial aspect of the conchal cartilage (i); (ii) base of pinna.

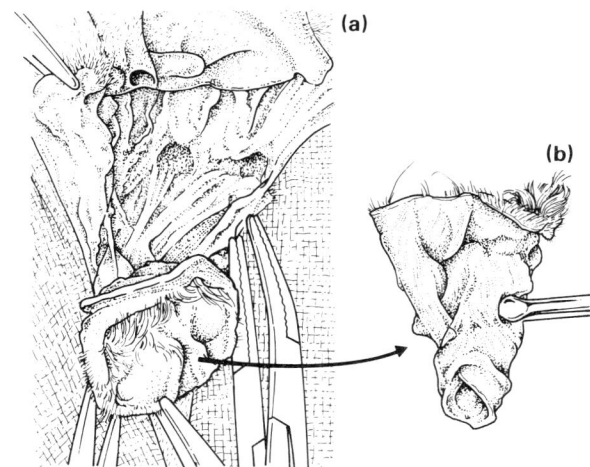

Fig. 2.4. (a) The conchal cartilage has been freed from the base of the pinna by cutting through cartilage; (b) the excised funnel of conchal cartilage.

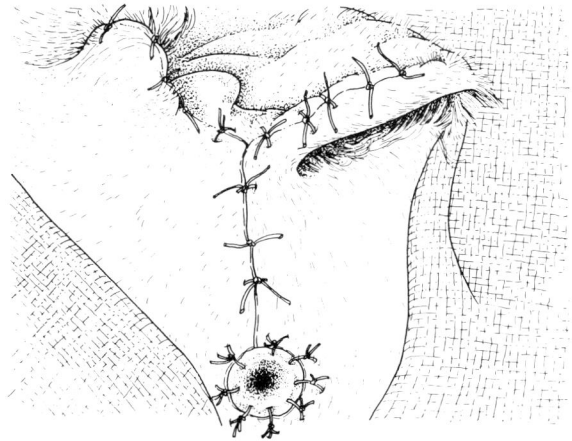

Fig. 2.5. The skin has been sutured to the rest of the horizontal part of the external auditory canal and the rest of wound closed by routine suturing.

Bulla osteotomy

Indications

The treatment of otitis media when bulla lavage is not appropriate or has failed.

Radiography is necessary to demonstrate changes within the tympanic bulla related to granulation, neoplasia or osteitis.

Equipment

A routine surgical set, plus bone drill, bone chisel, bone forceps, hammer and currette.

Technique

The patient is positioned in dorsal recumbency with the neck supported. The skin is incised medial to and parallel with the digastric muscle. The incision is centred over the tympanic bulla, which is located immediately medial to the muscular process of the mandible or the great cornu of the hyoid bone. The incision needs to be 5–8 cm in length according to the patient size to allow adequate exposure of the bulla. The subcutaneous tissues and the underlying mylohyoid muscle are incised, and blunt dissection between the digastric muscle laterally and the styloglossus and hypoglossus muscles medially will expose the tympanic bulla (Fig. 2.6). This is a difficult dissection, and damage to the hypoglossal nerve and the internal maxillary blood vessels is always possible if care and patience are not practiced. The knob of the bulla can be palpated through the tissues, and its frequent palpation will ensure that the dissection is in the right plane. The bulla is opened by either using the bone drill to penetrate its cavity and enlarging the hole using fine bone forceps, or a suitably sized bone chisel and hammer can be used to expose the cavity. The bulla is thoroughly curretted and aspirated, or else as much of the diseased bone as possible is removed (Fig. 2.7). A drainage tube may or may not be inserted, and the muscle, subcutaneous tissue and skin layers are closed in the usual manner.

Postoperative care

Routine antibiosis.

Possible complications

Otitis interna with a loss of hearing and balance are possible if the vestibule is damaged. Horner's syndrome is due to damage of the sympathetic nerve trunk.

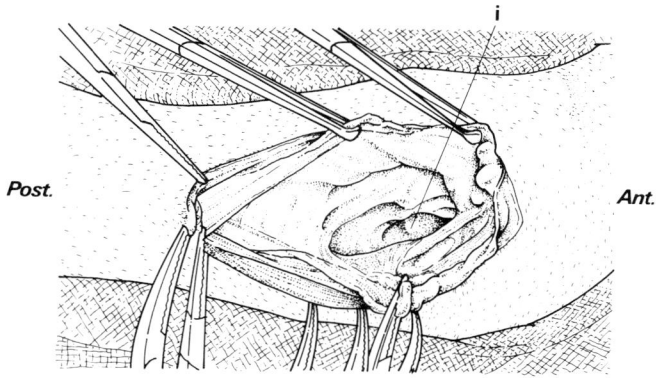

Fig. 2.6. Exposure of the tympanic bulla (i).

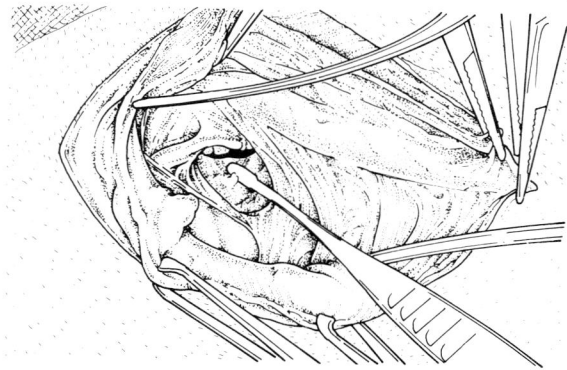

Fig. 2.7. Currettage of the tympanic bulla.

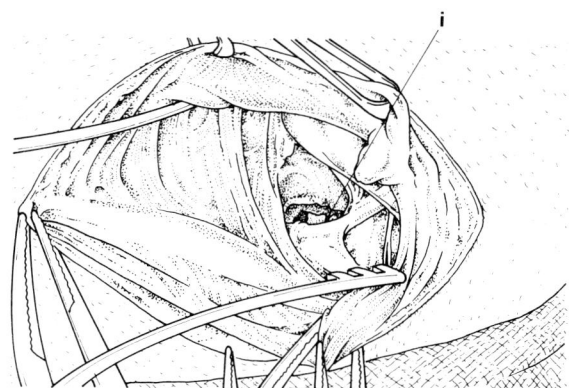

Fig. 2.8. The open tympanic bulla (i).

Rhinotomy

Indications

Rhinotomy is of diagnostic value when radiography is unable to specify between chronic rhinitis and early neoplastic change. It is used in the treatment of chronic bacterial, fungal or viral rhinitis by turbinate ablation, and in the removal of nasal polyps.

Equipment

A routine surgical set, plus small curved handsaw or an air-driven or power saw.

Technique

The patient is positioned in sternal recumbency, and the facial hair removed to the rami of the mandibles and the posterior limits of the frontal sinuses. It is essential that a cuffed endotracheal tube is used, and to further reduce the possibility of the aspiration of blood the nasopharynx should be packed off with gauze swabs. The skin is incised in the midline from the frontal sinuses to the anterior edges of the nasal bones (Fig. 2.10). Several large blood vessels are exposed at the anterior end of the incision, and these should be ligated before the rhinarium is incised. All subcutaneous and periosteal haemorrhage must be controlled before the nasal cavity is opened. Using the saw the rhinarium is incised to one side of the midline, and the incision is continued through the nasal and frontal bones to the posterior limit of the skin incision, parallel with the nasal septum (Fig. 2.11). A second incision, parallel with the first incision, involves the nasal premaxillary, maxillary and frontal bones (Fig. 2.13). A third incision across the rhinarial cartilage between these two incisions allows the bone flap to be hinged upwards on the frontal bone (Fig. 2.14). This bone is then cut across so that the bone flap can be removed in entirety (Fig. 2.14). The bone flap should be as wide as possible to allow the adequate manipulation of instruments within the nasal cavity. The removal of the flap allows inspection of the frontal sinus, the ethmoturbinate mass and the maxilloturbinates.

Polyps are easily removed, and unilateral turbinectomy performed using currettage and aspiration. Bilateral turbinectomy is effected by breaking down the nasal septum. When turbinate material has been removed, the nasal chamber(s) should be packed off with sterile gauze bandaging to control haemorrhage and prevent emphysema (Fig. 2.15).

The nasal cavity is closed using a simple interrupted suture pattern and absorbable sutures. This repair should be as air-tight as possible to prevent emphysema occurring. The skin is closed in the usual way (Fig. 2.16).

Postoperative care

Routine or specific antibiosis is maintained for as long as is indicated. Following turbinectomy the nasal packing is removed 5 days postoperatively.

Possible complications

Haemorrhage can be significant, and intravenous fluids/blood volume expanders should be given as routine. Subcutaneous emphysema will occur if the subcutaneous repair is inadequate. Turbinectomy can be complicated by new bone growth which can result in inspiratory dyspnoea.

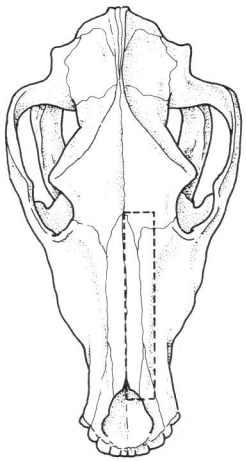

Fig. 2.9. The area of bone removed during rhinotomy. It includes the nasal bone an parts of the premaxilla, maxilla and frontal bone.

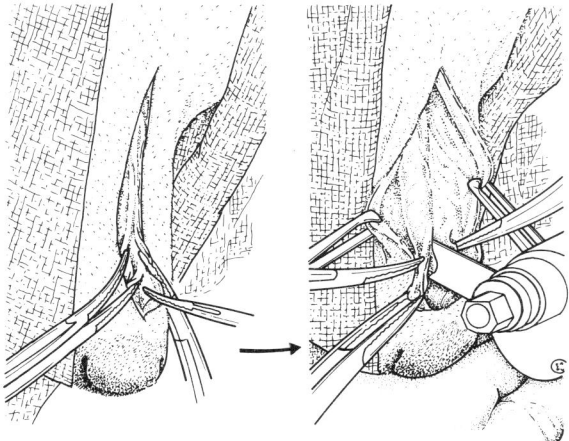

Fig. 2.10. The midline skin incision extending from the frontal sinuses to the anterior edge of the nasal bones. Blood vessels just posterior to the rhinarium should be ligated.

Fig. 2.11. An air saw is being used to cut into nasal bone parallel with and to one side of the nasal septum.

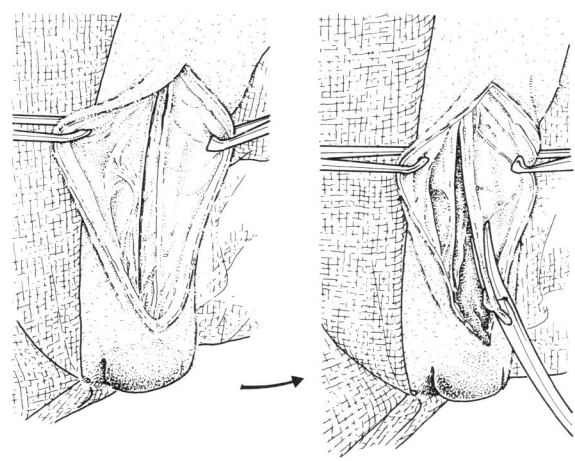

Fig. 2.12. The two parallel cuts have been completed.

Fig. 2.13. The bone flap is freed from the rhinarial cartilage and hinged upwards on the intact frontal bone.

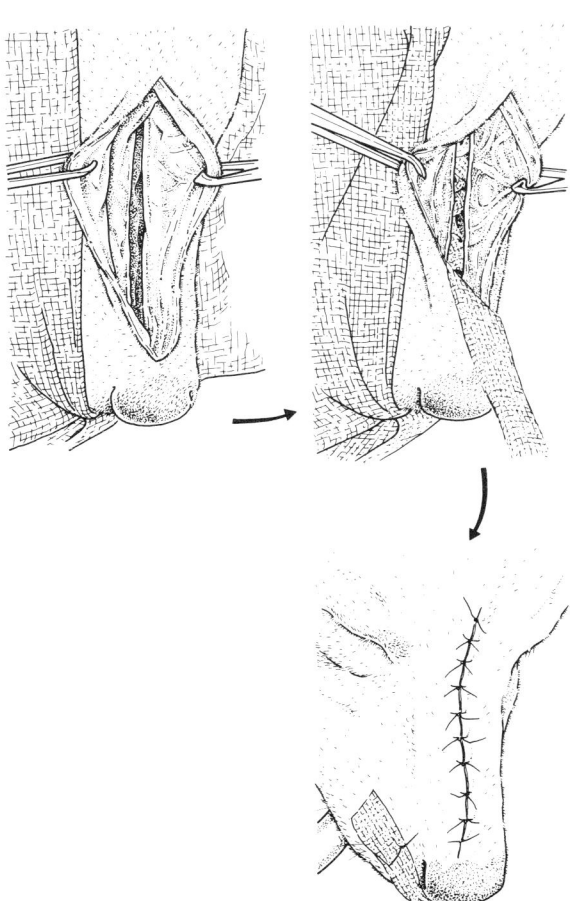

Fig. 2.14. The bone flap has been removed in entirety by cutting across its attachment to the frontal bone.

Fig. 2.15. A sterile gauze bandage is packed into the nasal cavity to occlude all the dead space, the end of the bandage being drawn through the nostril before closure.

Fig. 2.16. The wound is closed using subcutaneous and cutaneous single interrupted sutures. The end of the gauze bandage is sutured to the skin.

Soft palate resection

Indication

Inspiratory dyspnoea due to a relative overlength of the soft palate, usually in the brachycephalic breeds.

Equipment

Long-handled curved dissection scissors (Metzenbaum), long-handled rat-tooth forceps, long-handled suture forceps, tongue forceps and a dental gag.

Technique

The patient is positioned in sternal recumbency with the jaws held open using a dental gag. The maxilla is either supported by an assistant or suspended between two drip stands. The normal soft palate should not extend beyond the posterior limits of the tonsillar crypts, and it should just contact the epiglottis with the neck in moderate extension (Fig. 2.17). Adrenaline may be infiltrated along the palate margin to reduce possible haemorrhage, but invariably it produces tissue distortion and may predispose to inaccurate surgery. The pharynx is packed off with gauze swabs and a cuffed endotracheal tube is used to prevent the inhalation of blood. The soft palate is grasped at the mid-point of its free margin (Fig. 2.18), and the scissors are used to remove the excess tissue from first one half and then the other (Figs 2.19 and 2.20). Haemorrhage is likely to occur laterally, but such haemorrhage is easily controlled if the cut edge of the palate is sutured using a simple interrupted pattern and absorbable suture material (Fig. 2.21).

Postoperative care

Routine antibiosis should be continued for 5 days, and corticosteroid therapy will reduce the amount of pharyngeal oedema that can occur. Very small dogs are perhaps best maintained with an indwelling tracheotomy tube for the first 5 days following surgery.

Possible complications

An insufficient resection of the palate will still leave the patient with dyspnoea, whilst an overzealous resection will lead to the entry of food and fluids into the nasal cavity during swallowing. A posterior rhinitis may occur.

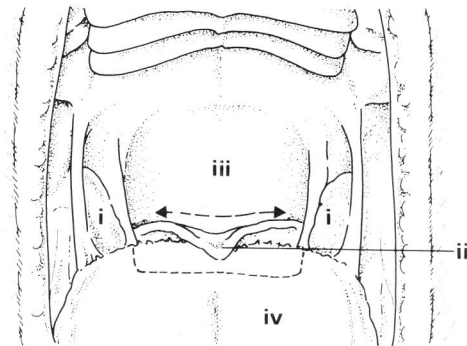

Fig. 2.17. Schematic representation of the amount of soft palate to be removed in the resection (dotted lines). The soft plate being 'sucked' into the laryngeal vestibule during inspiration. (i) Tonsils; (ii) epiglottis; (iii) soft palate; (iv) tongue.

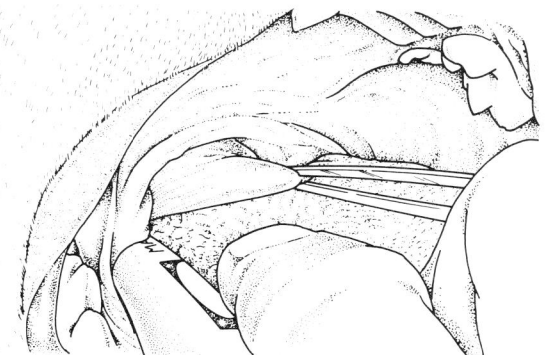

Fig. 2.18. The soft palate is gripped at the midpoint of its free margin using Allis tiisue forceps or rat-tooth dressing forceps.

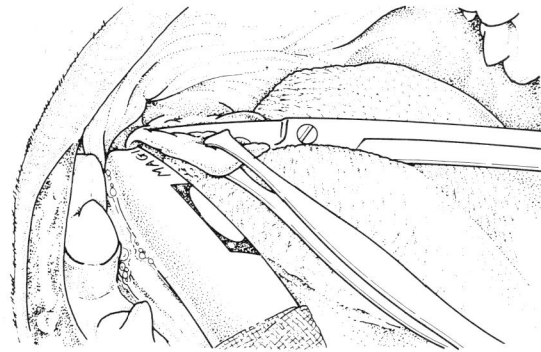

Fig. 2.19. The excess tissue from the right half of the palate is being removed using a Metzenbaum scissors.

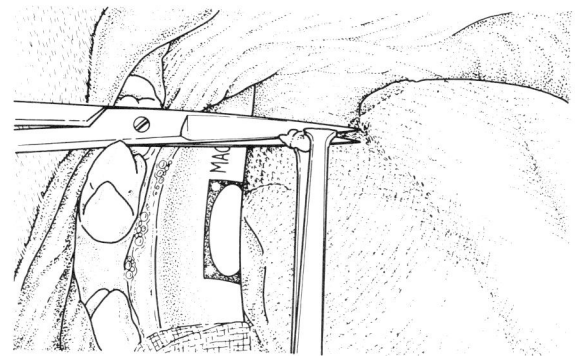

Fig. 2.20. The forceps have been repositioned on the palate, and the excess tissue from the left half is being removed.

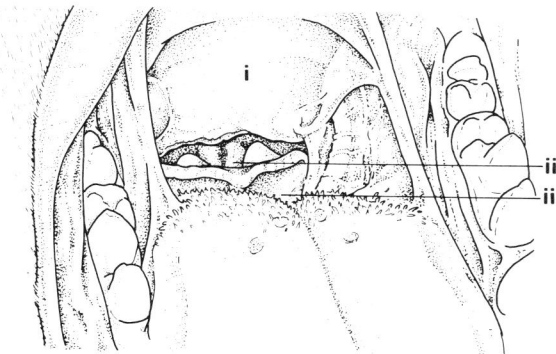

Fig. 2.21. The resected palate, the edge of which should be closed using simple interrupted sutures. (i) Soft palate; (ii) arytenoid cartilages; (iii) epiglottis.

Cleft soft palate repair

Indication

The treatment of rhinitis as the result of congenital cleft or insufficiency of the soft palate. A midline cleft may be seen in association with a midline cleft of the hard palate. Unilateral or bilateral hypoplasia in which the 'cleft' or 'clefts' are to one or both sides of the midline are notoriously difficult to repair.

Equipment

Long-handled curved dissection scissors (Metzenbaum), long-handled rat-tooth forceps, long-handled suture forceps, tongue forceps and a dental gag.

Techniques

1 The repair of the midline cleft is best achieved by removing the edges of the cleft to produce four flaps, and then closing the defect using two lines of simple interrupted sutures. The posterior line of closure, the nasopharyngeal mucosa and the nasal half of the palate should utilize absorbable suture material with the knots being tied on the oral side (Fig. 2.23). The anterior line includes the oropharyngeal mucosa and the oral palatine tissue, and either a permanent or an absorbable suture material may be used (Fig. 2.24).

2.25) can be achieved by either utilizing tonsillar crypt tissue or flap of pharyngeal mucosa. The former is preferred because it is simpler and there is less postoperative oedema (Fig. 2.26).

The tonsil is removed in the usual way and the lateral border of the palate is split along the edge of the cleft to create anterior and posterior flaps (Fig. 2.26b). The posterior crypt wall tissue is roughened and sutured to the posterior palatine flap using absorbable suture material in a simple interrupted pattern. The anterior crypt wall tissue is similarly prepared and sutured to the anterior palatine flap using either an absorbable or a permanent suture material (Figs 2.26c and 2.27).

3 The repair technique for bilateral hypoplasia involves the union of the central 'uvula' of soft palate to the two tonsillar crypts in two operations.

Postoperative care

Swallowing puts stress upon the suture lines, and the use of a pharyngostomy tube can help, particularly in the repair of unilateral or bilateral hypoplasia.

Routine antibiosis is maintained for 7 days, and corticosteroid therapy will reduce the postoperative oedema.

Possible complications

Wound breakdown is common, and the owner should be aware of this possibility before surgery is embarked upon.

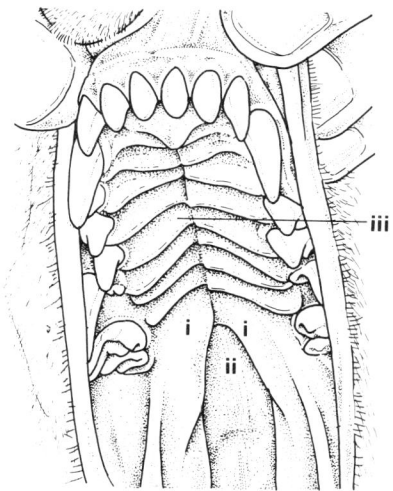

Fig. 2.22. Midline cleft of the soft palate. (i) The two halves of the soft palate; (ii) the nasopharynx; (iii) the hard palate.

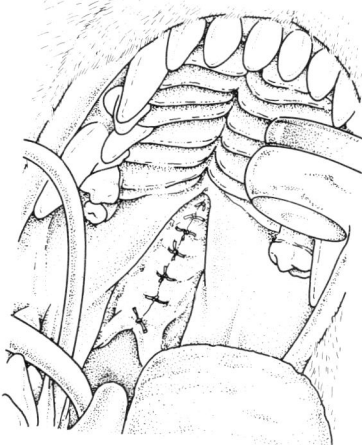

Fig. 2.23. The edges of the cleft have been split to produce posterior and anterior flaps of soft palate. The posterior (nasal) flaps have been sutured in the midline.

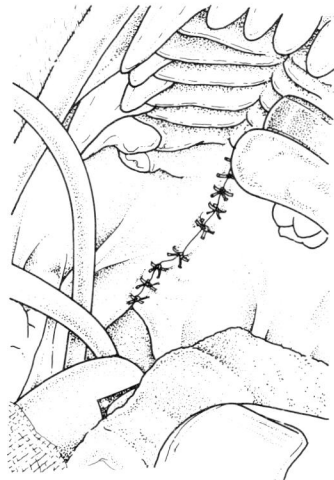

Fig. 2.24. The anterior (oral) flaps of soft palate have been sutured in the midline to complete a second level of repair.

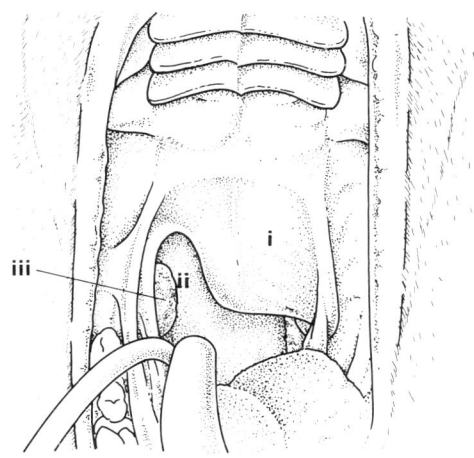

Fig. 2.25. Unilateral (right) hypoplasia of the soft palate. (i) Normal soft palate; (ii) the nasopharynx being viewed through the cleft in the palate; (iii) the right tonsil.

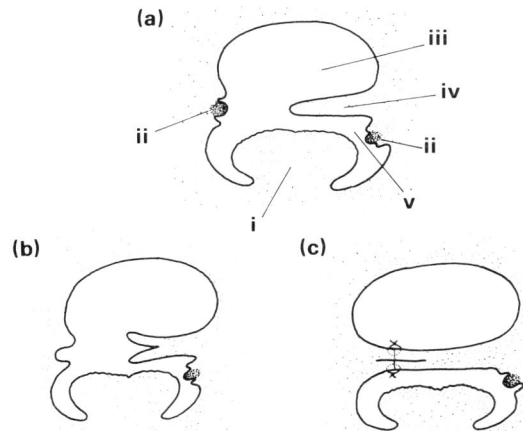

Fig. 2.26. Schematic representation of the repair technique. (a) Dorso–ventral section of the pharynx. (i) Tongue; (ii) tonsils; (iii) nasopharynx; (iv) palate; (v) oropharynx. (b) The right tonsil has been removed, and the edge of the palate has been split into dorsal (posterior or nasal) and ventral (anterior or oral) flaps. (c) The dorsal palatine flap has been sutured to the dorsal (posterior) tonsillar crypt wall and the ventral palatine flap has been sutured to the ventral (anterior) crypt wall.

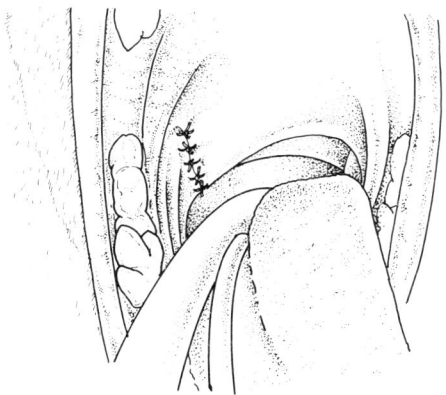

Fig. 2.27. The completed repair, the palatine tissue having been sutured to the right tonsillar crypt.

Resection of the sublingual/submandibular salivary gland complex

Indication

The treatment of cervical and sublingual mucocoeles.

Equipment

A routine surgical set.

Technique

Most salivary mucocoeles are the result of saliva leaking from the sublingual salivary gland or duct. Contrast radiography will specify the exact site of leakage, but the removal of the sublingual/mandibular salivary gland complex on the affected side provides the clinician with a simple effective method of treatment. The mandibular gland is rarely involved in mucocoele formation but it and the sublingual gland are resected as one because the two are so closely attached, and attempts to remove only the sublingual gland would damage the mandibular gland.

The patient is positioned in dorsal recumbency with the neck supported and the head rotated to present the salivary gland complex uppermost. The complex can be palpated easily at the angle of the jaw (Fig. 2.28), and a 4–6 cm skin incision exposes its fibrous capsule. The superficial maxillary vein lies dorsal to the complex, and the linguofacial vein is ventral. Blood vessels enter the complex on its dorsomedial aspect, and during the subsequent dissection these vessels should be ligated and transected. The capsule is opened, and the mandibular gland first is dissected free, traction being applied laterally (Fig. 2.29). As the dissection proceeds downwards and forwards the posterior part of the sublingual gland is freed and both the sublingual and the mandibular ducts will be seen running anteriorly between the masseter and the digastric muscles (Fig. 2.30). More traction is applied to the gland complex and the polystomatic portions of the anterior part of the sublingual gland are dissected free (Fig. 2.31). The dissection is continued as far forwards as possible, and the ducts are then either ligated and transected, or traction applied to the anterior limit of the exposed ducts pulls the tissue free. The wound is closed to obliterate the dead space with absorbable interrupted suture, and the subcutaneous tissue and skin are repaired in the usual way.

The mucocoele is simply drained by stab incision, and rarely should skin resection for the cervical swellings prove necessary.

Postoperative care

Routine antibiosis.

Possible complications

Although removal of the tiny anterior portions of the sublingual gland is not essential, further mucocoele formation can occur if parts of the mandibular or the posterior portion of the sublingual gland are left.

Bilateral leaks do occur to occasionally confuse both owner and surgeon.

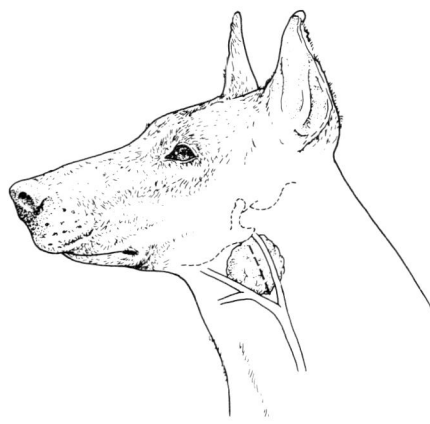

Fig. 2.28. The position of the left submandibular and posterior sublingual salivary gland complex.

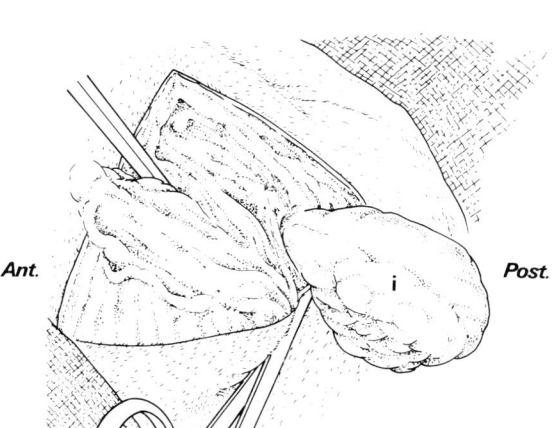

Fig. 2.29. The capsule has been opened and the conjoined salivary glands dissected free (i).

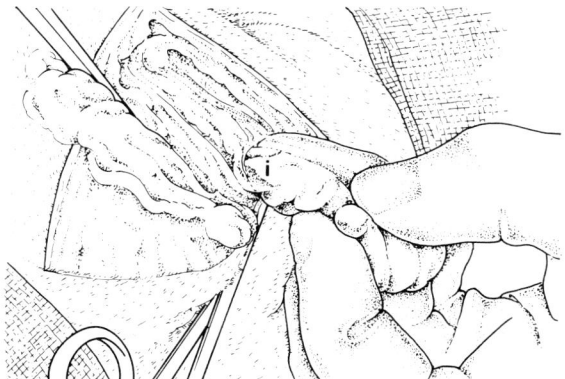

Fig. 2.30. Traction is applied to the gland complex, and blunt dissection reveals the anterior (polyostomatic) of the sublingual gland (i).

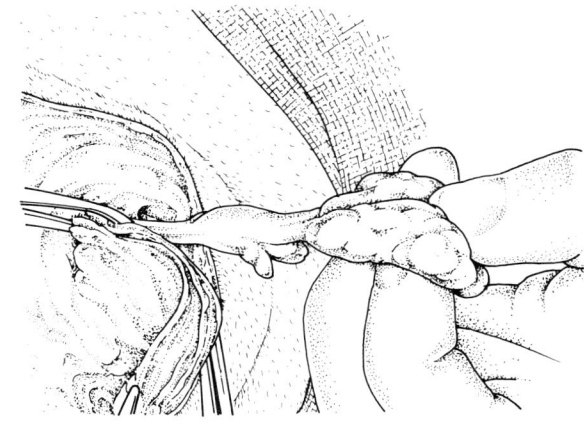

Fig. 2.31. The anterior parts of the sublingual gland and the ducts from both the sublingual and the submandibular glands are being dissected free.

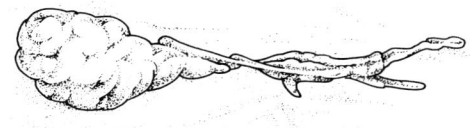

Fig. 2.32. The excised submandibular and sublingual gland complex together with their respective ducts.

Cricopharyngeal myectomy

Indication

The technique is used in the treatment of cricopharyngeal achalasia, in which inability of the cricopharyngeal sphincter to relax does not allow the passage of food from the pharynx to the oesophagus.

Equipment

A routine surgical set, plus a West's retractor.

Technique

The patient is positioned in dorsal recumbency with the neck supported and stomach tube is passed into the oesophagus. A midline skin incision from the anterior larynx to the thoracic inlet exposes the sternohyoid and sternocleidomastoid muscles, and the ventral trachea together with the intubated oesophagus are exposed by midline dissection through this muscle mass (Fig. 2.33). The sternohyoid muscles are retracted laterally, the left one being transected if necessary at the level of the larynx to expose the left sternothyroid muscle (Fig. 2.34). This muscle is then transected at its insertion on the lateral aspect of the thyroid cartilage of the larynx to expose the left thyroid gland and the recurrent laryngeal nerve (Fig. 2.35). The anterior part of the thyroid receives several small branches of the cranial thyroid artery, and these are ligated and cut. The larynx is then grasped and rotated to the right to expose the dorsal oesophagus and the cricopharyngeal muscle mass (Fig. 2.36). The presence of the stomach tube helps to identify the oesophagus and provides support for the production of the myotomy wound. A midline incision through the dorsal cricopharyngeal and oesophageal muscles exposes the oesophageal mucosa, and by lifting and separating the muscle mass from the mucosa laterally, part of the muscle mass 4 or 5 cm in diameter is removed (Fig. 2.38). Actual myectomy wound is not sutured. Closure of the sterno-inability of the oesophagus to dilate in this area postoperatively. Haemorrhage is not a problem, and the myectomy wound is not sutured. Closure of the sternothyroid muscle is not necessary, but the sternohyoid muscles are sutured in the midline using 3-0 gut. The subcutaneous tissue and skin are closed in the usual way.

Postoperative care

Routine antibiosis is provided for 5 days, and the skin sutures removed at 10 days. Fluid food only is fed on the first day, but after that small solid meals are offered for the next 2 weeks. Normal feeding may then be instituted.

Possible complications

Puncture of the oesophageal mucosa must be avoided, and both haemorrhage and damage to the recurrent laryngeal nerve are obviated by careful surgery. Fibrosis and oesophageal constriction at the myectomy site will occur unless sufficient cricopharyngeal muscle is removed. Correction requires further myectomy.

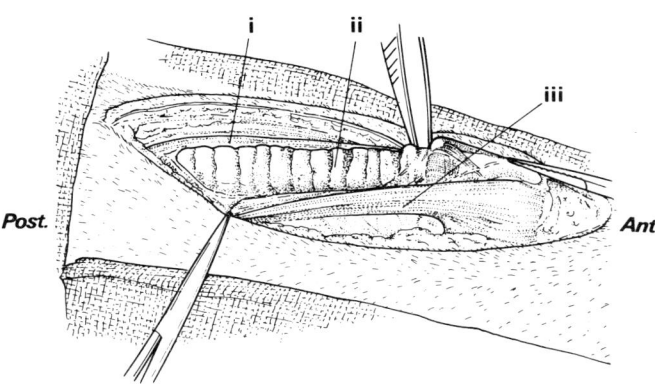

Fig. 2.33. A midline excision to expose the ventral surface of the trachea. (i) Sternohyoid and sternocleidomastoid muscles; (ii) trachea; (iii) left sternohyoid muscle.

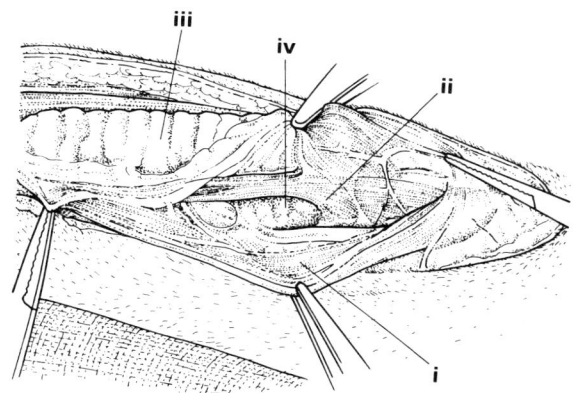

Fig. 2.34. The left sternohyoid (i) has been retracted (but not transected in this patient) to expose the left sternothyroid muscle (ii), (iii) shows the trachea and (iv) is the left thyroid gland.

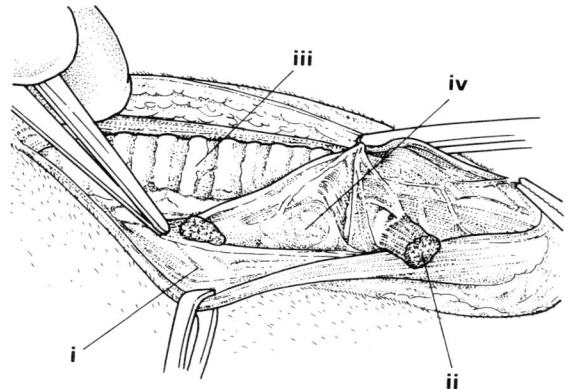

Fig. 2.35. The left sternothyroid muscle has been transected (ii); (i) is the left sternohyoid muscle; (iii) is the trachea and (iv) is the left thyroid gland.

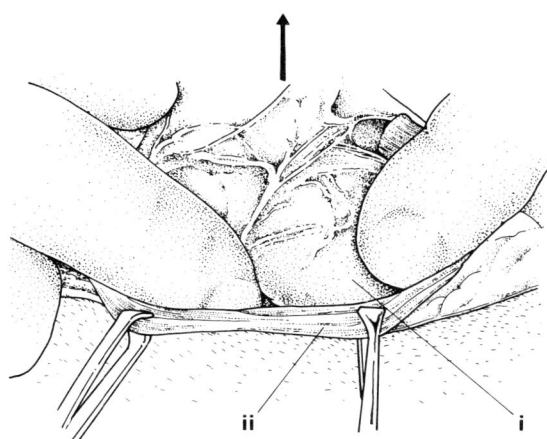

Fig. 2.36. Exposure of the cricopharyngeal muscle mass (i) by rotating the larynx to the right. (ii) The left sternohyoid muscle.

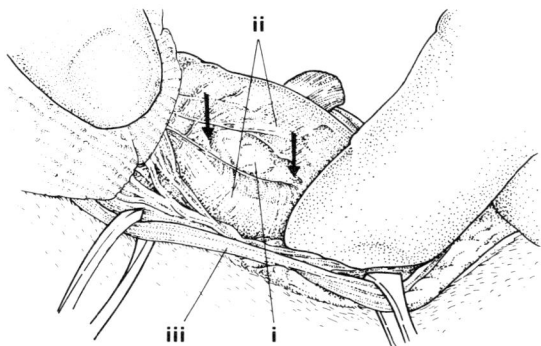

Fig. 2.37. The cricopharyngeal muscle (ii) has been incised (arrows) to expose the underlying oesophageal mucosa (i); (iii) is the left sternohyoid muscle.

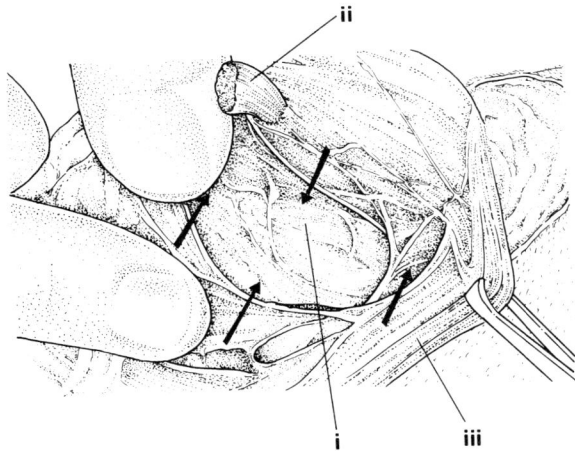

Fig. 2.38. (i) Part of the cricopharyngeal muscle has been excised (arrows) and the stomach tube may now be seen through the exposed oesophageal mucosa; (ii) is the proximal cut sternothyroid muscle stump and (iii) is the retracted left sternohyoid muscle.

Pharyngostomy intubation

Indications

The feeding of canine patients when food prehension, mastication or swallowing are impossible or contra-indicated. The indications are several:

1 To assist the repair of oesophageal wounds.
2 To maintain life until the patient with extensive cleft palate is mature enough for surgery.
3 During the postoperative phase of palate repair.
4 Pharyngeal paralysis.
5 Severe debility.
6 Mandibular fracture in which internal fixation is not possible.
7 Sublingual paralysis.

Equipment

A routine surgical set plus a dental gag. A rubber or polythene tube of 8 mm maximum external diameter is used, its length being determined by measuring the distance from the piriform fossa to the 10th costochondral junction via the acromion process (Fig. 2.39). (The tube should extend approximately 2.5 cm beyond the cardia.) The distal end of the tube should be rounded to reduce gastric irritation, and a suitable stopper is required for the proximal end of the tube. An alternative to a tube would be a Foley catheter.

Technique

The mouth is gagged open and a gloved index finger or the end of a pair of curved haemostat foreps is pushed into the piriform fossa in the pharynx (Fig. 2.40). The pharynx wall is tented out, and a 1 cm skin incision exposes this tissue. The site is sufficiently anterior to avoid the carotid or maxillary blood vessels and the hypoglossal nerve. The pharyngeal wall is then penetrated using either blunt or sharp dissection. The cranial end of the tubing is passed into the mouth and withdrawn through the pharyngostomy wound. The caudal end of the tube is passed into the mouth and pushed down the oesophagus (Fig. 2.41). If the Foley catheter has been used the cuff is inflated to prevent the tube bending on itself should the patient attempt to vomit postoperatively. The tube/catheter projecting from the pharynx is secured to the neck by retaining sutures and bandage. It can be left in position for weeks to months, and after its removal the pharyngostomy wound will heal without the need for suturing and without complication.

Postoperative care

It is always wise to check the position of the tube immediately postoperatively by radiography. Antibiotic cover is provided for 5 days, and daily cleansing of the wound continues until it remains clean. Liquidized food is fed four to eight times per day, 20 to 100 ml at a time depending on the size of the patient. The tube is capped between meals to prevent a back flow of gastric contents.

Complications

Too short a tube can result in regurgitation and ultimately oesophagitis, whilst too long a tube will promote vomition. Vomition can dislodge the tube should the skin fixation be inadequate. Blockage of the tube can occur.

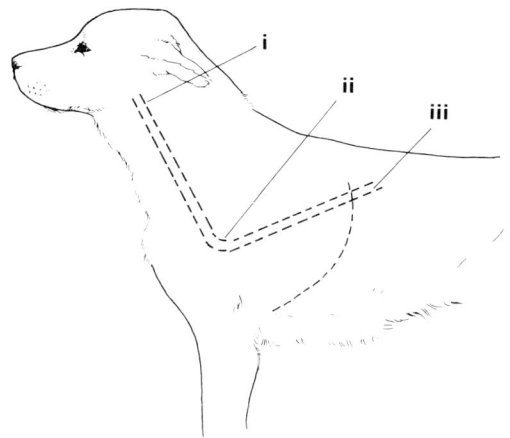

Fig. 2.39. The length of the tube. (i) Piriform fossa; (ii) acromion process; (iii) 10th costochondral junction.

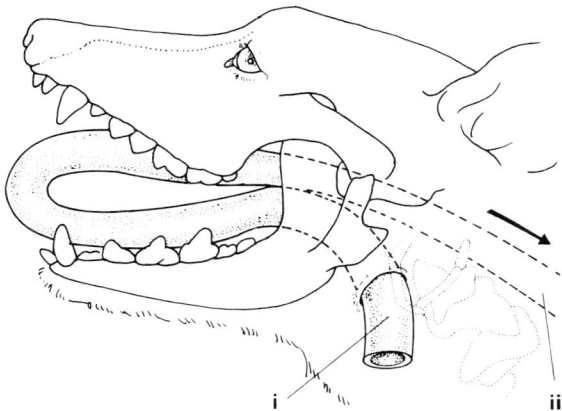

Fig. 2.41. The cranial end of the tube (i) has been passed from the piriform fossa through the incision to the exterior. The caudal end (ii) is passed down the oesophagus.

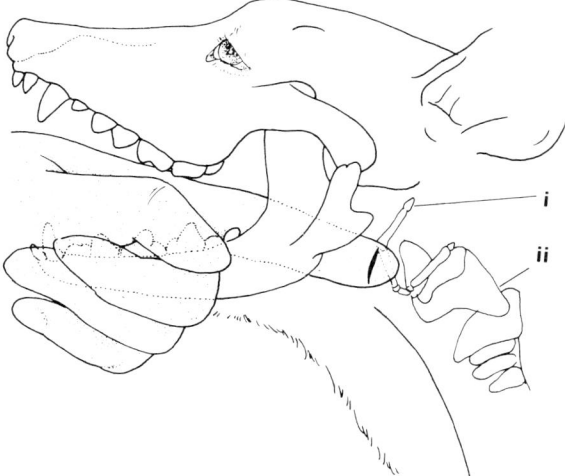

Fig. 2.40. A forefinger is placed into the piriform fossa, tenting it outwards prior to incision. (i) Hyoid apparatus; (ii) larynx.

Laryngeal cordectomy by laryngotomy

Indications

This technique is useful for reducing phonation in the dog (absolute debarking cannot be achieved surgically) and is considered by some authorities to be of value in reducing the degree of inspiratory dyspnoea due to laryngeal paralysis.

Equipment

A routine surgical set plus long-handled curved dissection scissors (Metzenbaum), long rat-tooth forceps and two Gelpi retractors.

Technique

The patient is positioned in dorsal recumbency with the neck supported. A ventral midline skin incision is made over the larynx and the proximal five tracheal rings to expose the paired sternohyoid muscles. These muscles are separated along their midline raphe to expose the ventral aspect of the larynx and the anterior trachea (Fig. 2.42). A simple scalpel incision between the third and fourth tracheal rings allows the insertion of a cuffed endotracheal tube to maintain anaesthesia. The cricoid and thyroid cartilages are identified, and the cricothyroid membrane is seen as a short, triangular, depressable structure filling the space formed by these cartilages. The overlying blood vessels should be ligated or cauterized to reduce post-operative filling and avoid haematoma formation. The cricothyroid membrane is incised along its midline, and the incision is continued anteriorly to separate the two wings of the thyroid cartilages (Fig. 2.43). The edges of the wound are retracted to expose the glottis and the vocal cords (Fig. 2.44). Each cord is completely excised, one point of the scissors being placed into the ventricle at the ventral insertion of the cord and the dissection being continued around the lateral limit of the cord to the vocal process (Fig. 2.45). Haemorrhage should be expected, and can be quite heavy if the branch of the laryngeal artery near the vocal process is sectioned. All bleeding must be controlled before the laryngotomy wound is repaired, for airway obstruction during the recovery phase can prove fatal. Both the thyroid cartilage and the cricothyroid membrane wounds are repaired using 2-0 absorbable suture material (polyglycolic acid, Dexon) in a simple interrupted pattern (Fig. 2.46). It is of no consequence if the suture material enters the lumen of the larynx, but the wound should be effectively sealed to prevent subcutaneous emphysema. The sternohyoid muscles are sutured in the midline, and the subcutaneous tissues and the skin are closed in the usual way.

Postoperative care

The patency of the laryngeal airway must be regularly checked, and corticosteroid therapy can be used to reduce possible laryngeal oedema and 'webbing'. Routine antibiosis is maintained for 1 week.

Possible complications

Postoperative haemorrhage must be avoided by suitable haemostasis at the time of surgery. Laryngeal oedema can be a problem in the smaller patient, and should be reduced by using corticosteroid therapy. 'Webbing' as the result of extensive fibrous tissue formation at the site of surgery can reduce the width of the airway, but again this can be controlled to some extent by using corticosteroid therapy for several days. This latter tends to be a problem in the patient with laryngeal paralysis, for 'webbing' occurs more extensibly in the absence of laryngeal movement.

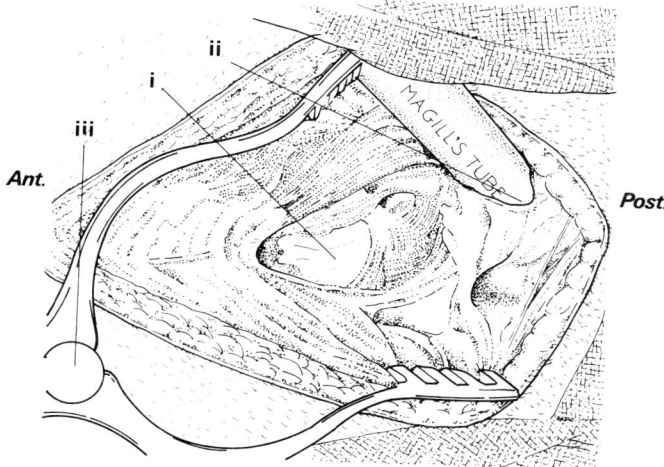

Fig. 2.42. A midline incision has exposed the ventral aspect of the larynx (i), and an endotracheal tube (ii) has been inserted into the trachea between the third and fourth rings; (iii) is the Gelpi retractor.

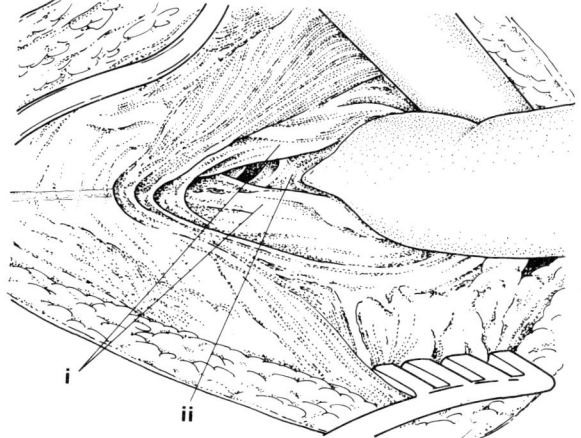

Fig. 2.43. The cricothyroid membrane has been incised along its length (a finger has been inserted through the cut membrane to indicate the incision) and the thyroid wings (i) have been split along their basal line of junction (ii).

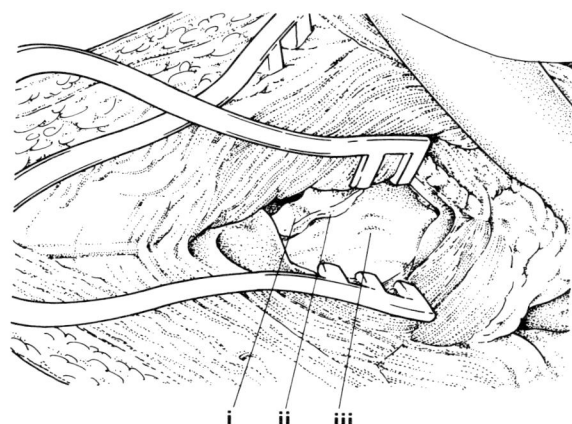

Fig. 2.44. A second pair of Gelpi retractors is used to hold the laryngotomy wound open. (i) The position of the left lateral ventricle; (ii) the left vocal cord; (iii) mucosa covering the left thyroid wing.

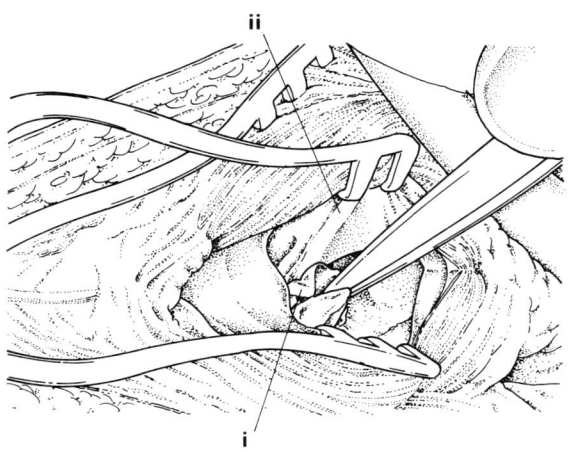

Fig. 2.45. The left vocal cord (i) is being removed by scissor dissection from the left thyroid wing (ii).

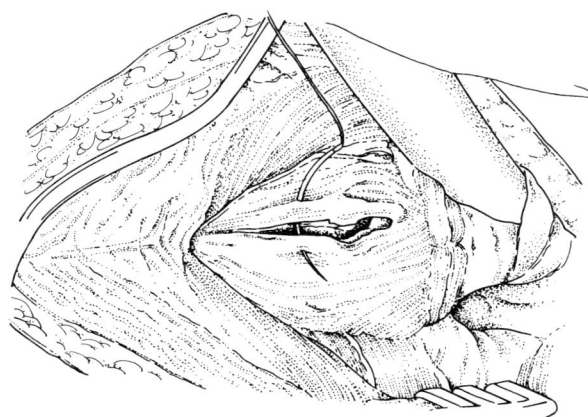

Fig. 2.46. Closure of the laryngotomy wound using 2-0 suture material.

Arytenoid lateralization

Indication

This recently innovated technique is proving to be of considerable value in the treatment of laryngeal paralysis in the dog. Bilateral cordectomy (page 78) can be complicated by postoperative 'webbing', but in arytenoid lateralization, sometimes referred to as the 'tie back' technique, the rima glottidis is held open by traction external to its lumen. An arytenoid cartilage is disarticulated from the underlying cricoid cartilage, and attached more posteriorly to the ipsilateral wing of the thyroid cartilage, thus abducting the attached vocal cord.

Equipment

A routine surgical set and no special instrumentation, although Metzenbaum scissors can be helpful in disarticulating the arytenoid cartilage.

Technique

The reader should familiarize himself with the structure of the laryngeal cartilages before attempting this technique (Fig. 2.47). The patient is positioned in lateral recumbency with the neck extended (either arytenoid cartilage may be moved). The skin is incised anteriorly at the level of the vertical ramus of the mandible, the incision extending posteriorly for approximately 8 cm at a level just below the external maxillary vein (Figs 2.49 and 2.50). The lateral aspect of the larynx is identified, and the overlying sheet of panniculus muscle is incised to display the thyropharyngeus muscle. This muscle 'wraps' around the body of the larynx, and it is incised along the length of the dorsal border of the wing of the underlying thyroid cartilage (Fig. 2.51). Scissors are then used to separate this wing of cartilage from the underlying cricoid cartilage, by disarticulating the caudally positioned cricothyroid articulation (Figs 2.48b and 2.51). The muscular process of the arytenoid cartilage is then identified, the overlying oesophagus being held away using suitable retractors. Careful scissor dissection is used to disarticulate the arytenoid from the cricoid cartilage (Fig. 2.48c), and the sesamoid band (cartilage) which lies between the two arytenoids in the midline is then sectioned (Figs 2.48d and 2.53). The arytenoid is now only attached to the laryngeal mucosa and the vocal cord. It is then positioned against the medial aspect of the caudal limit of the dorsal edge of the thyroid wing, and sutured into this position using a 0 or 2-0 braided steel mattress suture (Figs 2.48e and 2.54). The incision in the thyropharyngeus muscle is closed, and the subcutaneous tissues and skin are sutured in the usual way.

Both arytenoid cartilages may be 'tied back' in this way, but the author has witnessed no great benefit over the unilateral approach, and subsequent coughing has been more of a problem.

Postoperative care

The patency of the larynx should be checked whilst the patient is still anaesthetized, but hospitalization need only be for a 24 h period. Routine antibiosis is employed for 7 days.

Possible complications

Severe dyspnoea may arise in the event of the inadequate anchorage of the arytenoid to the thyroid wing, but this complication will usually be seen within 7 days of surgery. A firm ankylosis between the two pieces of cartilage should be expected, and will result in a permanent rapid improvement in inspiration. Coughing related to an inability to close the rima glottidis during swallowing is not a common postoperative feature.

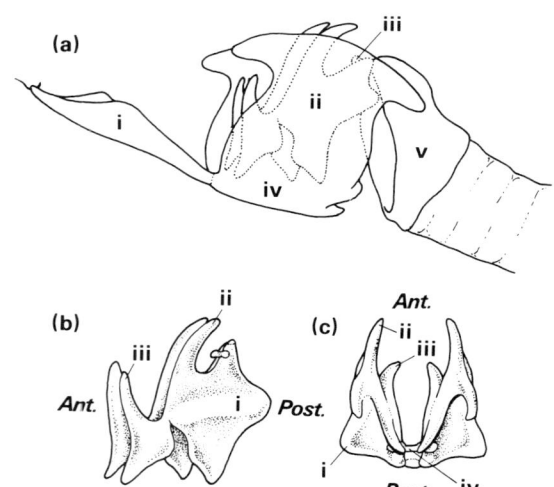

Fig. 2.47. Orientation of laryngeal cartilages. (a) Laryngel cartilages — lateral view: (i) epiglottis; (ii) Left arytenoid cartilage; (iii) position of sesamoid band; (iv) left wing of thyroid cartilage; (v) cricoid cartilage. (b) Arytenoid cartilages — lateral view: (i) muscular process; (ii) corniculate process; (iii) cuneiform process. (c) Arytenoid cartilages — dorsal view: (i) muscular process left; (ii) corniculate process, left; (iii) cuneiform process, left; (iv) position of sesamoid band (cartilage).

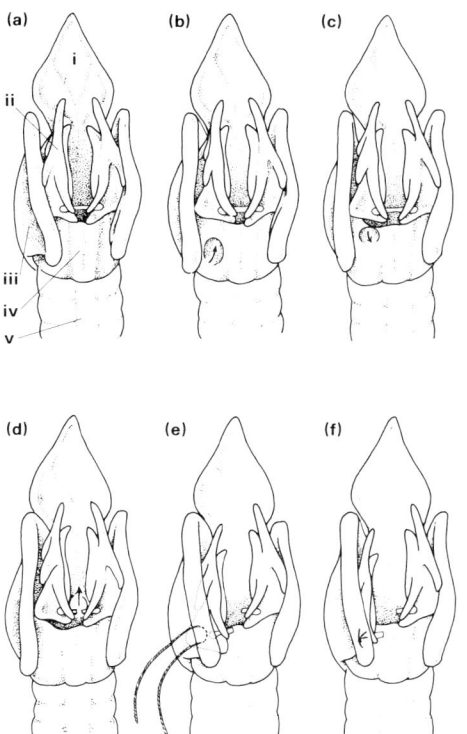

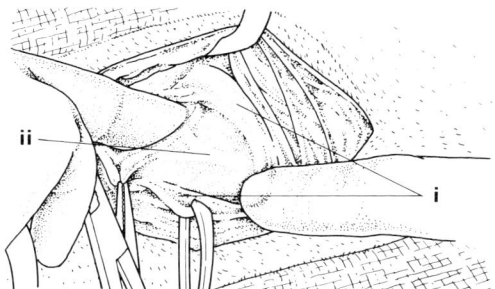

Fig. 2.51. The thyropharyngeus muscle (i) has been cut to expose the left wing of the thyroid cartilage (ii). A finger has been inserted medial to the wing of the thyroid, and the attachment of the distal part of the wing to the underlying cricoid cartilage is dissected using scissors.

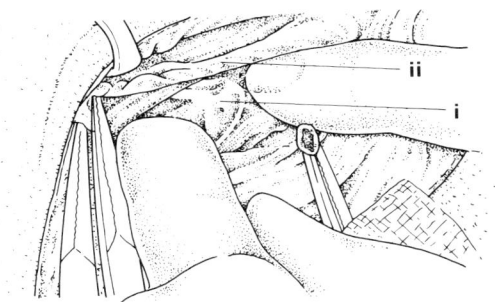

Fig. 2.52. The muscular process (i) of the left arytenoid cartilage is identified; (ii) is the oesophagus.

Fig. 2.48. Schematic representation of the technique—dorsal view of the larynx. (a) Before surgery: (i) epiglottis; (ii) left arytenoid cartilage; (iii) left thyroid wing; (iv) cricoid cartilage; (v) trachea. (b) The separation of the left thyroid wing from the cricoid cartilage. (c) The separation of the left arytenoid cartilage from the cricoid cartilage. (d) Section of the sesamoid band (cartilage). (e) Suturing the left arytenoid cartilage to the caudal aspect of the left thyroid wing. (f) The completed operation. operation.

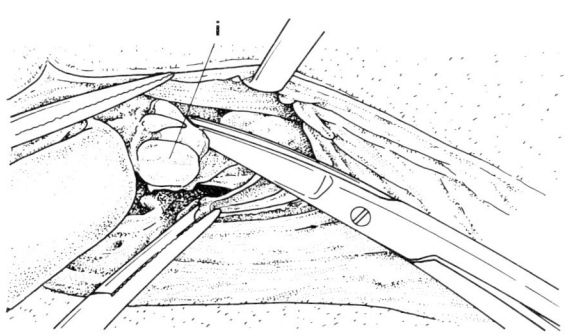

Fig. 2.53. The sesamoid band has been cut and the whole of the left arytenoid cartilage (i) is now mobile.

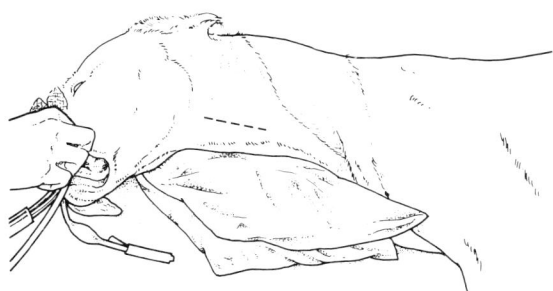

Fig. 2.49. The site of incision.

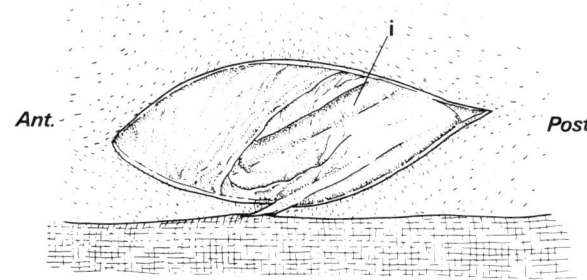

Fig. 2.50. Exposure of the left external maxillary vein (i).

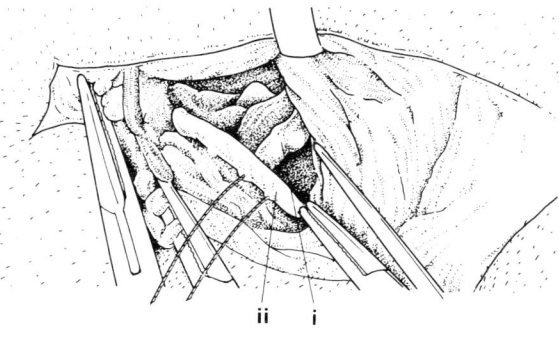

Fig. 2.54. The muscular process of the left arytenoid cartilage (i) is sutured to the caudal aspect of the left thyroid wing (ii).

Plication of the tracheal ligament

Indication

The treatment of tracheal collapse. This condition occurs usually in the smaller breeds of dog and is due to degeneration of the cartilagenous tracheal rings, the stretched tracheal ligament occluding the tracheal lumen during inspiration. A constant cough may be the only indication of the condition until severe inspiratory dyspnoea and collapse occur.

Equipment

A routine surgical set plus permanent suture material (2-0 silk).

Technique

The technique is only of value when the collapse has confined itself to the cervical trachea.

The patient is positioned in dorsal recumbency, and a ventral cervical midline incision through the skin and subcutaneous tissue from the anterior larynx to the thoracic inlet exposes the paired sternohyoid and sternocephalic muscles. The sternohyoid muscles are split along their midline raphe to expose the trachea, and blunt dissection around the length of the trachea (Fig. 2.55) allows it to be rotated to expose its dorsal surface (Fig. 2.56). Plication of the stretched tracheal ligament is obtained using several horizontal mattress sutures placed 0.5 cm apart. The bites should be large, the needle entering the tissue of the ligament just medial to tracheal rings. Ideally the tracheal lumen should not be entered. This suture pattern everts the tracheal ligament from the tracheal lumen, and draws the end of the cartilaginous rings close together to reform a lumen that is round in cross section (Fig. 2.57). The sternohyoid muscles are then sutured in the midline, and the skin and subcutaneous tissues repaired in the usual way.

Postoperative care

Routine antibiosis is used for 7 days, and several days corticosteroid therapy can help reduce postoperative oedema. Coughing should be suppressed and exercise limited for 10 days.

Possible complications

Collapse of the plication immediately postoperatively will result if the sutures are placed with excessive tension or very close together. Coughing can also lead to damage to the suture line.

Experience has shown that with the passage of time the plicated ligament will again stretch and the clinical signs of collapse will recur. However, this simple technique is easily performed, and repeated surgery can be as successful as the initial operation.

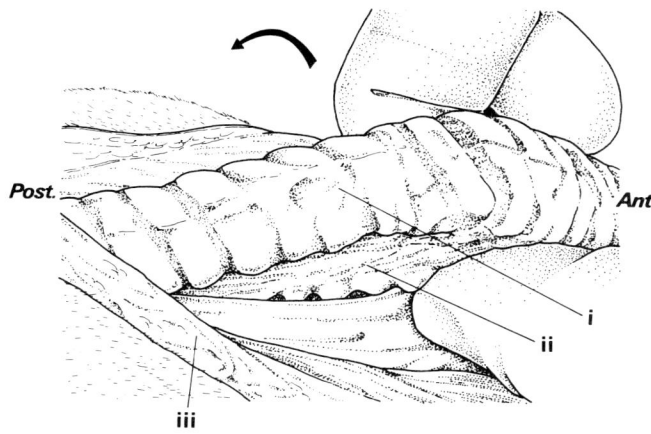

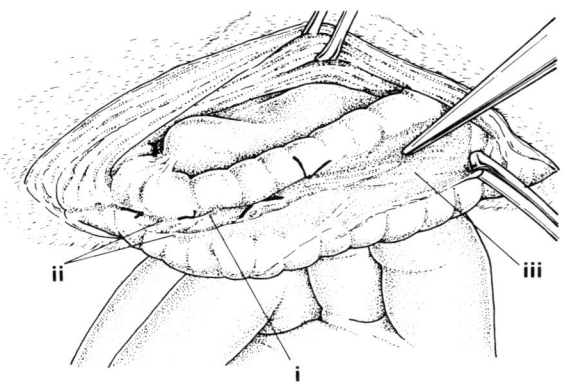

Fig. 2.57. The tracheal ligament is being plicated (i), drawing the ends of the rings together (ii). The ligament will be plicated at this point next.

Fig. 2.55. The trachea has been freed from the surrounding connecting tissue and is being rotated towards the right. (i) Left side of tracheal rings; (ii) stretched tracheal ligament coming into view; (iii) left sternohyoid muscle.

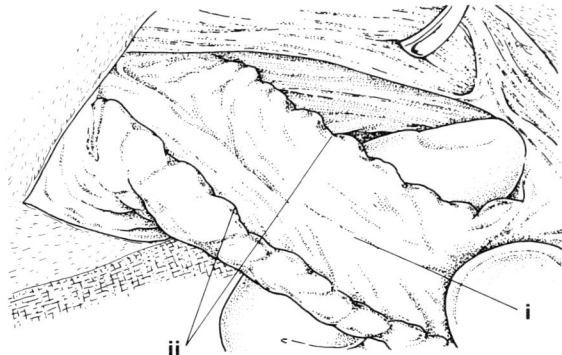

Fig. 2.56. The trachea has been rotated 180° to expose the stretched tracheal ligament (i); (ii) are the open ends of a cartilagenous ring.

Chapter 3
Thoracic Surgery

D. GARETH CLAYTON JONES

Thoracentesis (Chest drainage)

Indications

To empty the pleural cavity of either fluid or air, either as an acute procedure or over a period of days/weeks. Chest drainage may be a specific therapeutic procedure or a part of postoperative management following another procedure:

1 Air—pneumothorax.
2 Fluids—transudate, exudate, blood, pus, chyle.

Acute procedure

Equipment

A large bore intravenous type of cannula, approx. 10–14 gauge, a three-way tap, and a large syringe, 50 or 100 ml capacity. Local anaesthesia using fine 25 G needle.

Technique

Prepare the skin over the selected site; if an urgent procedure simply spray the area with surgical spirit and part the hair. Inject a small volume of local anaesthetic subcutaneously and scratch the skin surface with a needle point to indicate the area anaesthetized (Fig. 3.1a). Close the three-way tap. Insert the cannula horizontally and advance the point beneath the skin until it lies one interspace cranial to the point of skin entry (Fig. 3.1b). Tilt the cannula and needle vertically and insert it intercostally until it enters the pleural cavity. Quickly remove the needle and attach the closed tap to the cannula. Open the tap and aspirate using the large syringe (Fig. 3.1c). Empty the syringe after each filling by turning the tap. As the lungs will float on fluid and sink in air, use posture to assist with drainage (Fig. 3.1d). Moving the cannula horizontally may help to clear the end of fibrin tags or blood clots. On completion of drainage remove cannula, and as the skin wound does not overlay the intercostal puncture there will be no danger of pneumothorax.

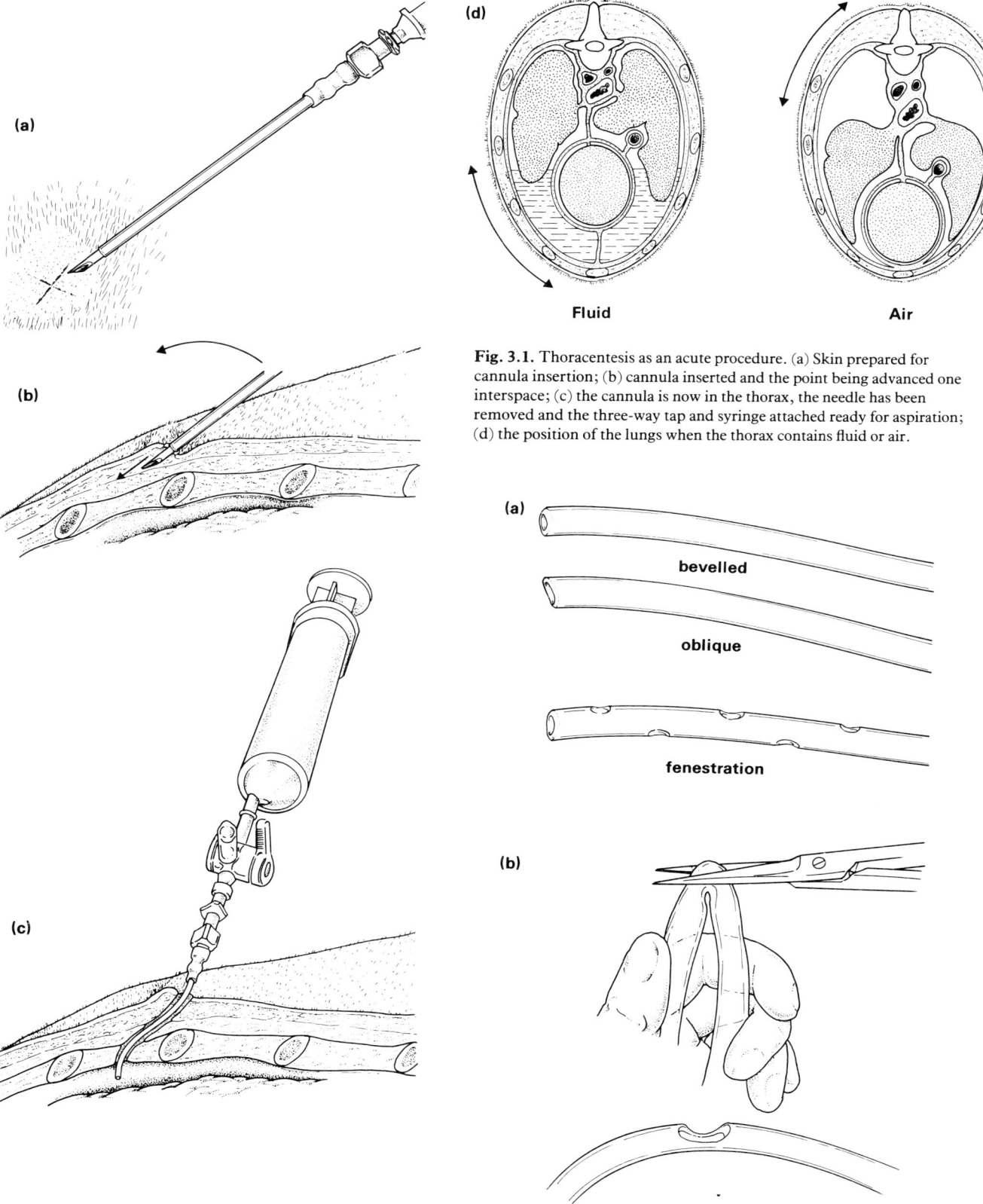

Fig. 3.1. Thoracentesis as an acute procedure. (a) Skin prepared for cannula insertion; (b) cannula inserted and the point being advanced one interspace; (c) the cannula is now in the thorax, the needle has been removed and the three-way tap and syringe attached ready for aspiration; (d) the position of the lungs when the thorax contains fluid or air.

Fig. 3.2. Chest drain during thoracotomy/or as a chronic procedure. (a) The end of the drain is either bevelled or oblique, and the drain is fenestrated; (b) the fenestrations are prepared by folding the distal end of the drain and cutting off the corners produced. The fenestrations should not be too deep, otherwise the drain may rupture.

During thoracotomy or as a more chronic procedure

Equipment

Scalpel with a No. 15 blade, a chest drain, a connector (prepared as in Fig. 3.2), a tubing clamp or tube forceps, Lahey cholecystectomy forceps, an underwater chest bottle and tube, or disposable aspiratory apparatus, a spigot to fit the chest drain, a needle holder, needles and suture material (0 silk or polyglycolic acid).

Technique

Make a small skin incision about 1–2 cm long, two interspaces cranial or caudal to desired site of chest drain. Close the chest drain with the tubing clamp and grasp the tube in the curved Lahey forceps with the open end of the drain just behind the forceps points. Insert the forceps points with the drain through the skin wound and pass it subcutaneously one or two interspaces until over the desired site of insertion, which should be one or two interspaces from any thoracotomy wound and *not* through the thoracotomy. Rotate forceps points 180° and plunge through intercostal muscles and pleura into the pleural cavity. While holding the drain with one hand, release the forceps with the other and withdraw them. If the drain is being inserted during surgery the forceps may be inserted from the surgical wound and the drain drawn inwards. An absorbable suture may be placed intrapleurally and tied lightly if needed to keep the drain *in situ* within the chest (Fig. 3.4). Ensure that all the fenestrations of the drain are within the pleural cavity, then tie the drain in place as shown (Fig. 3.4b).

Attach the connector to tube/bottle, and open the tubing clamp to begin aspiration as necessary.

When the drainage is complete, close the tubing clamp, remove the connector and insert the sterile spigot.

To remove the drain, cut the retaining suture loop (point X in Fig. 3.4b) so as to leave the purse string suture in place. Withdraw drain briskly, and the hole will close spontaneously (this can be assisted by using a skin adhesive spray, e.g. Nobecutane). As the skin wound and pleural wound do not overlay one another, the negative pressure within the pleural cavity tends to suck the skin surface down so as to plug the hole (Fig. 3.5).

Postoperative care

Keep the tube clean. A chest drain tube can transmit infection upwards. Sterilize the ends of the tubes and connectors with betadine before and after use. Clean the aspirator bottle with Hibitane as well as any connecting tubes and connectors. Remove the chest drain as soon as is possible, consistent with the clinical condition. For some simple surgical procedures this can be within 12 h, although a minimum of 24 h is preferable. If leakage is considerable then continuous drainage is needed, otherwise every 2–4 h is adequate. Chest drains should not be left in place for more than 7–10 days.

Possible complications

In the acute procedure the cannula/needle may damage the lung, and this can lead to pneumothorax or haemorrhage. Such punctures usually heal rapidly.

In the chronic procedure the following might arise:
1   Pleurisy due to an ascending infection.
2   Pneumothorax if the skin wound and pleural wound are over one another.
3   Loosening of the drain and its loss if not tied in place correctly.
4   Leakage if all the fenestrations of multi-hole drain are not in the plaural cavity.

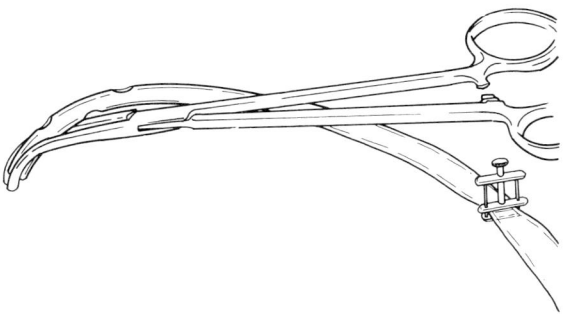

Fig. 3.3. The drain being held with the Lahey forceps ready for insertion with the tube clamp closed.

(a)

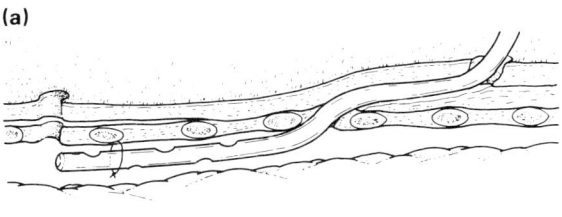

(b)

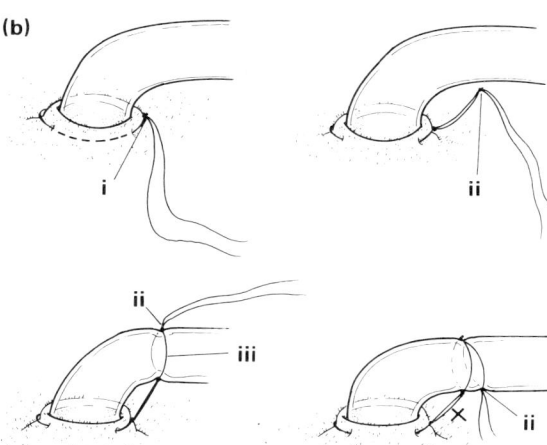

Fig. 3.4. (a) The drain *in situ* with all fenestrations inside the thorax. (b) The drain is retained in position using purse-string suture in the skin with a separate loop holding the tubing. (i) Purse string suture; (ii) reef knot plus one; (iii) suture material at right angles to long axis of drain.

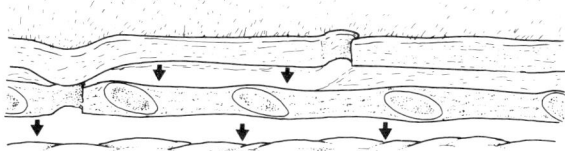

Fig. 3.5. Negative pressure closes the wound.

Thoracotomy

Indications

All operations on intrathoracic organs.

Equipment

A routine surgical set plus rib spreader (for large dogs use the Gosset retractor, for medium-sized dogs use the Gelpi or Travers retractor, and for small dogs use the West's retractor), long-handled scissors (Nelson/Metzenbaum) and bone-cutting forceps.

Technique

Several routes of entry may be used, the lateral intercostal, the transcostal, and the midline trans-sternally. For most indications, use the lateral intercostal route. Alternatively, a rib can be removed and the approach is then through the rib bed. The pleura and periosteum are somewhat fragile in dogs and the intercostal method provides adequate exposure and a good repair. The midline sternal split is useful for the repair of the ruptured diaphragm where entrapment or adhesion of abdominal viscera within thorax has occurred.

The hair is removed from the whole thoracic wall from R1 to R13 and from the spine to the sternum. The skin is finally prepared using Betadine solution after routine cleansing.

If the anaesthetist allows, raise the thorax on a small sandbag/folded cloths beneath the selected level of thoracotomy (Fig. 3.6). Fix the forelegs and hind legs, drawing them gently forwards and backward respectively. After draping count the ribs backwards to find the relevant rib space (as in Fig. 3.7) feeling for R1, and incise the skin over the selected intercostal space. The incision is extended through the cutaneous muscle until the belly of the latissisimus dorsi is seen in the dorsal wound (Fig. 3.8). This is incised across the line of its fibres, and the vessels within it are cauterized with diathermy. Beneath this can be seen the insertions of the m.serratus dorsalis, and these insertions over the relevant rib space are cut close to the ribs and elevated dorsally and cranially (Fig. 3.9).

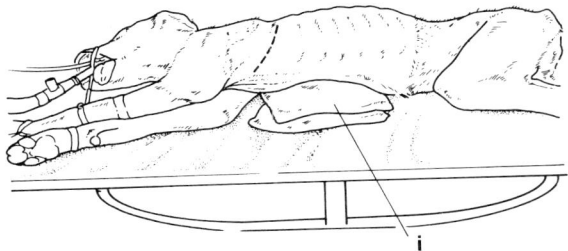

Fig. 3.6. Positioning the patient for thoracotomy. (i) Support to prop up the thorax.

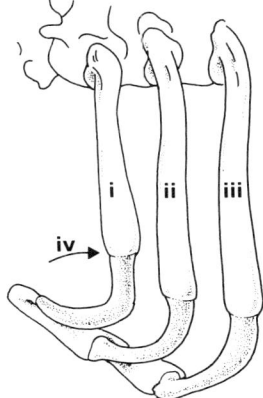

Fig. 3.7. Location of the site for incision. (i) Rib 1; (ii) Rib 2; (iii) Rib 3; (iv) the hooked part of Rib 1 is readily palpable.

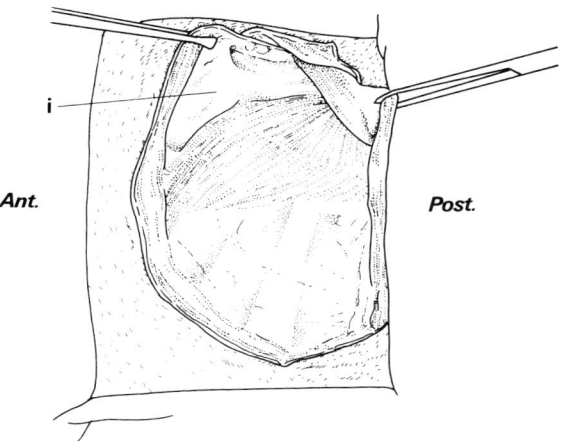

Fig. 3.8. Dissection of the thorax wall reveals the belly of latissimus dorsi (i).

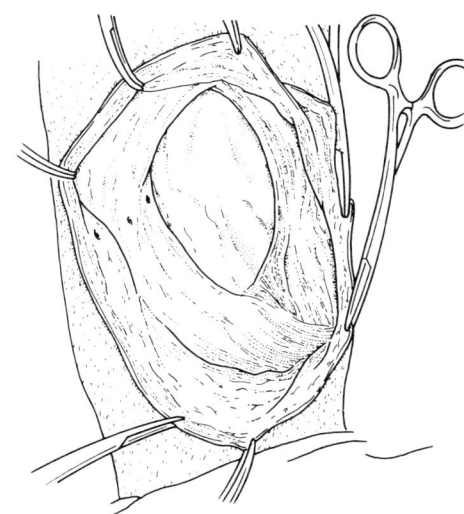

Fig. 3.9. Serratus dorsalis is incised to expose the external intercostal muscle.

In the ventral wound lie the insertions of external abdominal oblique muscles. These can be separated and cut away from the relevant ribs and retracted caudally and ventrally. The external intercostal muscle is then incised midway between the selected ribs with scissors, followed by the internal intercostal muscle and the pleura is then exposed. This is grasped with toothed forceps and then punctured with a scalpel point, taking care not to injure the lung beneath. The anaesthetist can assist here by not ventilating the patient for a moment. The initial puncture is then extended using blunt pointed scissors, taking care to avoid the caudal aspect of the rib and its associated intercostal vessels and the now deeper partly collapsed lung lobes. Care is needed where there are adhesions between the parietal and visceral pleura.

The chest cavity is then displayed by the insertion of a chest retractor of the correct size. Care should be taken to ensure that a lung lobe does not become trapped between the retractor and the thoracic wall, or that the points of the retractor do not damage the lung surfaces. If greater exposure is needed, the ribs on each side of the incision can be transected at one end and allowed to hinge back or forwards (Fig. 3.10).

The lungs may be retracted using a large folded swab moistened with saline or by means of a malleable retractor bent to shape and protected by a moist swab.

Prior to closure of the thorax, a chest drain is tied in place and attached to the chest bottle. The pack is then removed from beneath the chest. Encircling sutures are passed beneath the ribs using a curved needle, and the ends are left untied but clipped to a haemostat. These sutures may be of absorbable material or monofilament steel wire (about 20 G/0.7 mm). The first and third sutures are pulled up and held tight by the assistant, whilst the second suture is tied (Fig. 3.11). This procedure is repeated until the wound has been closed completely. The muscle incisions are then closed using polyglycolic acid interrupted sutures. The subcutaneous tissues and the skin are similarly closed, and the chest is bandaged lightly.

Repair of flail chest injury

Establish chest drainage, debride the wound and suture lung wounds. Absorbable sutures are passed around the adjacent intact ribs to attach the free area of chest wall to the nearest intact ribs (Fig. 3.11).

Postoperatively, a lightly padded bandage applied sufficiently firmly to keep the injured area in place, but not so tight as to cause restriction of respiration, will be of assistance.

Chest wall neoplasia

Tumours which originate in the ribs may be treated by radical excision. In general, such neoplasia tend to spread by local extension to involve neighbouring ribs. The neoplasia exhibit the 'iceberg effect' in that there is usually more neoplasm beneath the pleura and thus invading the pleural cavity than is visible as a subcutaneous mass.

Such tumours are best removed by excising the chest wall leaving a margin of about 2 cm on each side of the lesion. This will leave a roughly circular or oval defect. Haemostasis should be secured by diathermy and ligation. The rib ends in the centre of the lesion should be removed to create an oval excision with its long axis parallel with the ribs. For defects up to three or four ribs in width, closure can be effected by the application of encircling wires around the intact ribs and drawing the wires up to close the defect as far as possible. Remaining areas of leakage are closed by suturing of the overlying muscles and soft tissues.

Where such a defect cannot be closed then a patch of polypropylene gauze mesh (Marlex) can be applied over the area and attached using either Dexon sutures or nylon sutures to the neighbouring ribs. A final seal is obtained by regrowth of the soft tissues into the substance of the mesh. Recent work suggests the use of an omental graft to repair the defect.

Postoperative care

A postoperative chest drain is essential.

Possible complications

Failure to adequately drain the chest of fluid or air for a sufficient time. A chest drain should be kept in place for a minimum of 24 h in most cases.

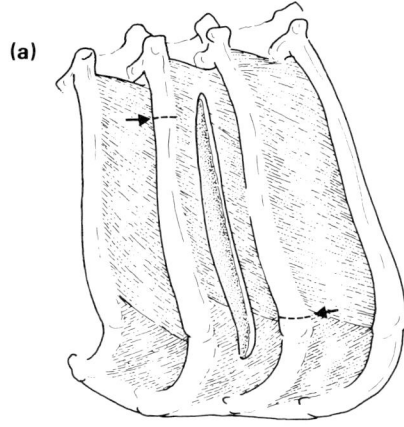

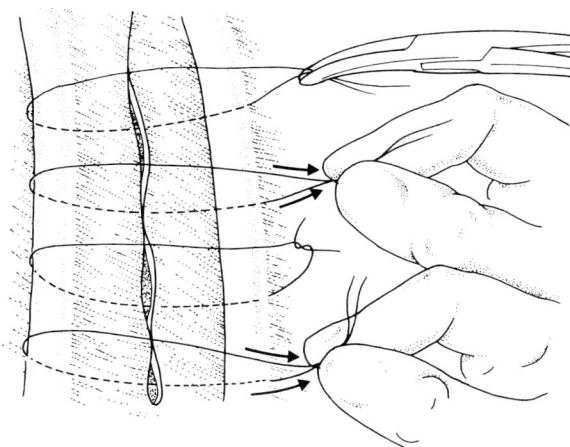

Fig. 3.11. Closure of the thorax.

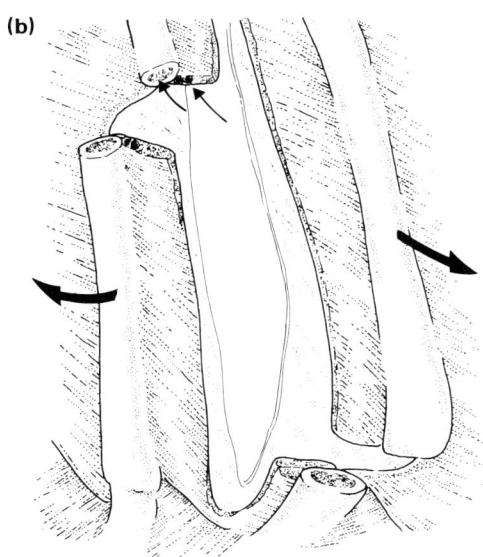

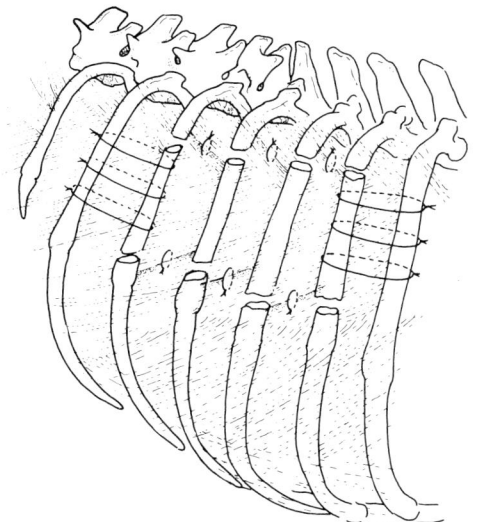

Fig. 3.12. Repair of the flail chest injury.

Fig. 3.10. Transection of ribs to allow greater exposure of the thoracic cavity. (a) The rib anterior to the intercostal section is cut using bone cutters near its proximal end, whilst the rib posterior to the section is cut towards its distal end (arrows). (b) The cut ribs may be then hinged on their attachments to allow greater exposure. The intercostal arteries must be ligated, and should the rib ends bleed then bone wax may be applied.

Surgery of the patent ductus arteriosus and the persistent right aortic arch

Indications

As title.

Equipment

A routine surgical set plus malleable retractors, Lahey forceps, ductus clamps (if division and suture is contemplated), Crafoord clamps (to cross-clamp the aorta and pulmonary artery if haemorrhage occurs), and a gauze pack 22.5×22.5 cm or 30×30 cm.

Technique

The thorax is opened routinely at the left fourth or fifth intercostal space. The apical and cardiac lung lobes are gently retracted caudally, using a moist pack and malleable retractor as described before. The branches of the vagus and phrenic nerves should be identified and gently mobilized and retracted using silk sutures. The ductus can be identified by palpation between the ascending aorta and the pulmonary artery, and the ligamentum arteriosum by the area of constriction caudal to a preplaced oesophageal bougie or stomach tube.

The mediastinal pleura is opened over the abnormal vessel and any bleeding points are occluded using diathermy. The pericardial sac may also be incised to aid identification of the structures, a long vertical or cruciate incision being used. Any bleeding points in the pericardium should be sealed by diathermy as they can be the source of considerable haemorrhage.

The ductus or ligament is then dissected gently—until its cranial border, between it and the ascending aorta can be seen (Fig. 3.13). (The use of a blunt point scissors or haemostat is safest.) Care should be taken not to damage the recurrent laryngeal nerve or the thoracic duct. The Lahey forcep is then passed caudal to cranial beneath the ductus, gently advancing the points into the space cranial to the vessel. Gentle persuasion and patience will normally allow the points to appear without penetration of the thin medial wall of the ductus or pulmonary artery. A moistened loop of 0 or 1 silk is then grasped by the fold and drawn caudally (Figs. 3.14 and 3.15). The loop is then cut, the relevant ends identified, and the two sutures tied so as to lay two ligatures across the ductus (Fig. 3.16). To aid manipulation of the great vessels a piece of soft rubber tubing (Paul's tubing) passed around the descending aorta caudal to the ductus will allow movement of the aorta and facilitate separation of the ligatures.

Transection of the patent ductus is unnecessary and revascularization is unusual following double ligation. Some authors recommend dissection of the roots of the aorta and main pulmonary artery prior to dissection of a ductus in order to allow the application of vascular clamps in the event of a major haemorrhage following perforation of the ductus. This technique is not normally carried out by this author. The pericardial sac should *not* be sutured but rather allowed to remain widely open to facilitate drainage of any pericardial effusion that may result.

The same method is used for persistent right aortic arch except that the ligament is usually longer and may safely be divided between the ligatures (Fig. 3.16). The vascular remnants and the adherent mediastinal pleura should be gently dissected from the lateral and ventral oesophagus until a stomach tube will readily pass the point of obstruction.

Closure of the chest with a chest drain is performed routinely, and the chest drain can normally be removed in 24 hours.

Postoperative care

There are no particular features other than the care involved in the nursing of a routine thoracotomy patient. A slowing of the heart rate after closure of a PDA is usual, and is due to a reduced left-sided load: it may be noted at surgery. The murmur disappears immediately and if it reappears this indicates failure of the ligation.

Possible complications

No specific complications follow this procedure although revascularization of the ductus is recorded in the literature, resulting in a return of the murmur and symptoms.

Failure of full return of normal function of the oesophagus is not unusual in the vascular ring obstruction and oesophageal stricture may occur at the site of the previous obstruction. The presence of the large diverticulae in the oesophagus cranial to the obstruction site is a poor sign, and plication of these dilated areas should be considered.

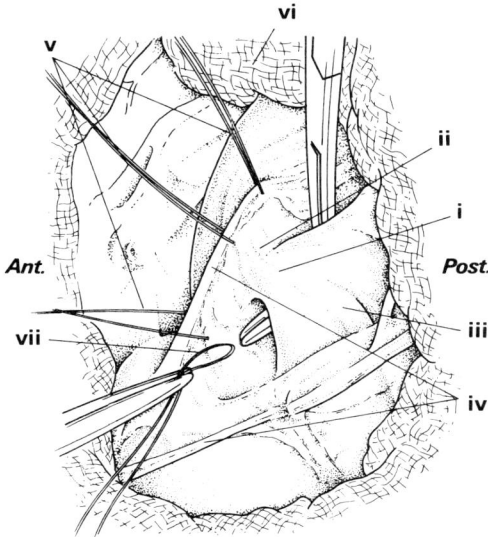

Fig. 3.13. Repair of patent ductus arteriosus. (i) The patent ductus; (ii) the aorta; (iii) the dilated pulmonary artery; (iv) vagus and phrenic nerves; (v) traction sutures; (vi) gauze packing; (vii) silk loop.

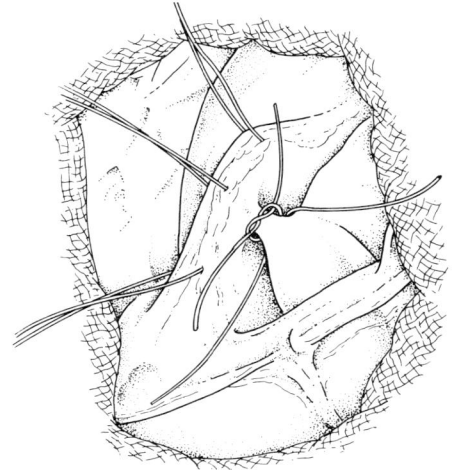

Fig. 3.15. The loop is cut and tied as two ligatures.

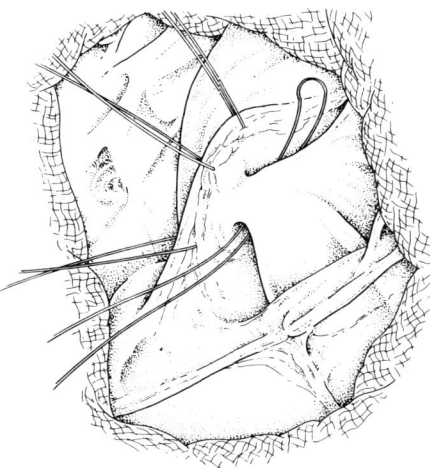

Fig. 3.14. The silk loop has been passed beneath the persistent ductus.

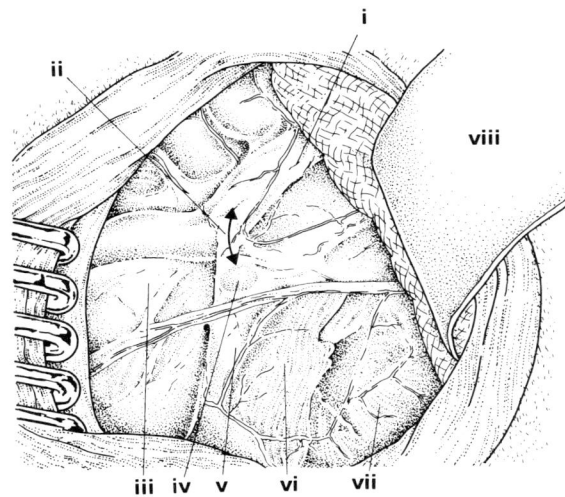

Fig. 3.16. Persistent right aortic arch. (i) Aorta; (ii) the ligamentum arteriosum; (iii) distended oesophagus; (iv) lymph node; (v) pulmonary artery; (vi) left auricle; (vii) left ventricle; (viii) malleable retractor.

Transsthoracic oesophagotomy

Indications

Foreign body obstruction of the oesophagus where manipulative removal *per os* cannot be performed. Perforation of the oesophagus, and diverticulum or tumour formation.

Equipment

A routine surgical set plus malleable copper retractors, an aspirator and stomach tube, long-handled suturing instruments and grasping forceps for f.b. removal (e.g. large Allis' forceps, haemostats or whelping forceps). Spare drapes, gloves and suturing instruments are also required.

Technique

The site for thoracotomy is selected by calculating the level of the foreign body by means of a stomach tube or oesophageal bougie, or by counting ribs over the obstruction as seen radiographically. Generally the incision will not be behind the seventh intercostal space. The left side is usually opened as described for thoracotomy.

The lung lobe overlaying the involved oesophagus should be retracted. The diaphragmatic lobe is attached caudally and deeply by a thin fold of pleura and this should be incised so as to allow reflection of the lobe forwards. Retraction can be accomplished by using a large folded and rolled gauze swab of 22.5×22.5 cm or 30×30 cm depending on the size of the dog. The swab should be thoroughly wetted with warm saline prior to insertion. If necessary the swab should be held in position using a malleable copper retractor bent to fit the incision. It should be remembered that all swabs, packs and instruments put into the thorax will compress the lung space available and thus reduce the available lung volume for the anaesthetist. Care must also be taken to ensure that the retractor in particular is cushioned by the swab and positioned so that the end of the instrument does not occlude a major blood vessel.

Once the involved area of oesophagus is exposed, dissection around the vagal trunks should be carried out using a long-handled curved scissors and a long, fine-toothed forceps. Once freed from the mediastinal pleura, long lengths of moistened No. 1 silk should be passed around the nerves and the ends of the threads held in a small haemostat. These sutures should then be used to retract the nerves away from the oesophagus to allow exposure and incision of the mediastinum.

The wall of the oesophagus may then be grasped using a Babcock forceps cranial and caudal to the lesion and the oesophagus tented up gently to avoid leakage. Suction through an oesophageal stomach tube *per os* may remove fluids cranial to the obstruction although fluids caudal to the obstruction will remain. The remaining area of the thorax should be adequately covered with almost dry swabs to absorb any spillage and to protect the pleural cavity.

Spare drapes may also be applied over the wound edges to protect any exposed tissues from contamination. In many cases the oesophageal wall exhibits extensive oedema and the organ is relatively fixed within the mediastinum. It is better to try and avoid contamination and leakage by adequate packing, than to damage the oesophagus and its tenuous blood supply, with instruments and violent traction.

The oesophagus is incised along its length, where possible through healthy tissue. A small incision made first, aspirated and then enlarged is better than one bold incision that allows a flood of contamination. Gentle diathermy will secure haemostasis of the larger bleeding points. The foreign body is removed using a suitable grasping forceps which should be discarded together with the foreign body. Following aspiration of the lumen the epithelial lining should be inspected for signs of perforation and if necessary sutured from the incision, using Dexon, such that the knots lie within the lumen.

The oesophagus is then closed in two layers of interrupted sutures using absorbable material with the knots of the epithelium layer lying within the lumen (Fig. 3.17). The sutures in the muscular layer may be holding soft, oedematous, weak tissues and should be tied with care.

The packs should then be removed, the spare drapes and instruments discarded, and gloves changed and the pleural cavity washed with saline and aspirated. Local antibiotic solution should be instilled and the chest drain should then be inserted. The lung pack is then removed and using clean instruments the chest should be closed.

Postoperative care

Routine antibiosis is required.

Where any serious damage of the oesophagus is suspected a pharyngostomy tube should be placed and the patient fed by pharyngostomy for about 7 days. The chest drain can be removed after 2 days in most cases unless effusion is seen. The patient should not be allowed solid food for up to 10 days depending on the degree of damage and nature of the surgery.

Possible complications

These are mainly a mediastinitis following contamination of the region either at surgery or following a perforation. High levels of antibiotic and perhaps re-operation and placement of the chest drain close to the site may be required although the prognosis is often poor in such cases.

Perforation of the oesophagus at the suture line may cause a pneumothorax to develop. This can be sudden and may well be fatal.

Failure of the oesophageal function because of oedema initially and because of stricture formation later are also possible. Pharyngostomy will allow the former to settle, while bougienage or oesophageal resection may be required for the latter.

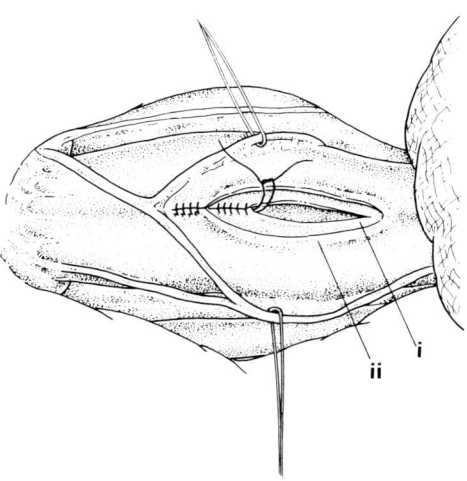

Fig. 3.17. Suturing the oesophagus. (i) Epithelium; (ii) muscular layer.

Rupture of the diaphragm

Indications

Diaphragmatic rupture occurs as both a congenital and an acquired defect.

Equipment

A routine surgical set plus long-handled scissors, rat-tooth forceps and needle holder. Malleable retractors, bone cutting forceps and large gauze packs are also required.

Technique

A midline laparotomy will allow adequate exposure of all diaphragmatic lesions. Anaesthesia should be induced after as much preparation of the patient as possible and the surgeon and instruments should be prepared for immediate surgery if an anaesthetic crisis should arise. Following induction the patient should lie with the ruptured side downmost and the trunk slightly sloping to the tail during preparation. Positioning on the operating table should be head high/tail low to allow some gravitational reduction of the rupture, with the animal in dorsal recumbency. The preparation of the animal should include the caudal half of the *thorax* to allow for sterile placement of a chest drain and extension of the incision into the sternum if necessary.

Following a rapid routine midline laparotomy from xiphoid to umbilicus the abdominal organs should be removed from the thoracic cavity as soon as possible to give the anaesthetist maximum lung space. Any portion of displaced abdominal content that can be moved should be moved. If the rupture wound has become cicatrized and stenosed the defect in the diaphragm should be immediately enlarged towards the sternum using a blunt straight scissors until the entrapped contents can be released (Fig. 3.18). If adhesion of abdominal contents to the thoracic contents has occurred and gentle traction and manipulation will not release them the midline incision should be extended forwards with bone-cutting forceps to involve the caudal mid-sternum, thus allowing the adhesions to be seen and divided under direct vision. Engorged lobes of liver are best returned by *elevation* gently using a finger through the enlarged defect (Fig. 3.19). Rupture of the liver lobes is likely if traction is used.

Once the thorax is empty of the abdominal contents then the anaesthetist has no ventilation problems and repair of the defects both acquired and created, can take place in an unhurried manner. Grasp the deepest edges of the rupture using Allis forceps and ensure then that any adhesions to the liver are divided. Cover the exposed abdominal contents with a large moist pack—this will normally give adequate retraction to retain abdominal contents in the abdomen. A chest drain should now be inserted and tied in place *before* beginning to repair the diaphragm. Aspirate any free pleural fluid, then the diaphragm defect may be repaired using silk sutures.

Lay all the sutures and hold the ends in haemostats, then tie the sutures at the end. This allows better exposure during placement of the final sutures. Begin with the deepest sutures and work up towards the ventral midline. A simple interrupted pattern is preferable as any small leaks readily become sealed by the abdominal organs following closure of the laparotomy. A continuous suture is not so easy to adjust and the last few throws are inserted blindly. Care should be taken not to pass sutures through the vena cava where it passes through the diaphragm nor to occlude it by tight suturing. It is easier to pass the needle from abdomen to thorax, and using a curved needle the lung can be protected from the needle point by the fore finger of the other hand. Where the diaphragm is torn from the costal margin, sutures should be passed around a suitable nearby rib.

Following closure of the rupture, the abdominal contents should be rearranged, swabs counted and Allis forceps applied to the wound edges. Elevation and crossing of these forceps will facilitate the closure of the abdomen even in longstanding cases of diaphragmatic rupture, as well as the judicious use of muscle relaxants.

Where the sternum has been split, suturing of the rectus abdominis muscle will usually be adequate although if an extensive incision has been made wire or absorbable sutures may be needed around the affected segments of sternum.

In peritoneal pericardial hernia the defect is central and may be quite large. The defect can usually be closed by suturing although some tension may be noted. Where such a defect cannot be closed or where a defect exists in a diaphragmatic rupture, polypropylene mesh may be applied to the defect with interrupted sutures of silk to form a repair.

Recent work suggests the use of an omental graft for the repair of such defects.

Postoperative care

Pain and pressure of the abdominal contents may restrict respiration in the early period following surgery. Analgesia should be used carefully so as not to compromise the blood pressure. The chest drain is normally not required beyond 24–48 h unless many adhesions have been divided, but a minimum period of 24 h is sensible as some apparently simple cases can produce large effusions in the early postoperative period.

Possible complications

Intestinal function should be checked, as vascular lesions resulting in ileus or necrosis may be encountered if rough handling or incorrect repositioning has occurred.

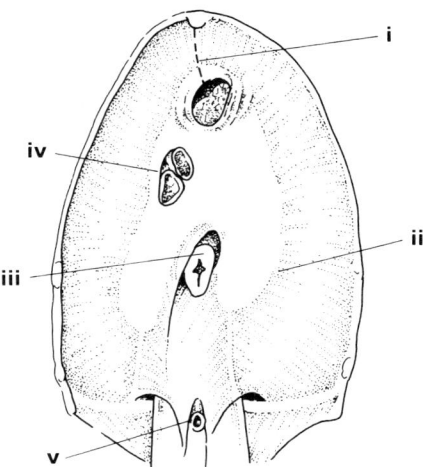

Fig. 3.18. Enlarging a cicatrized wound. (i) Cut to the middle to enlarge; (ii) diaphragm, abdominal side; (iii) oesophagus; (iv) posterior vena cava; (v) aorta.

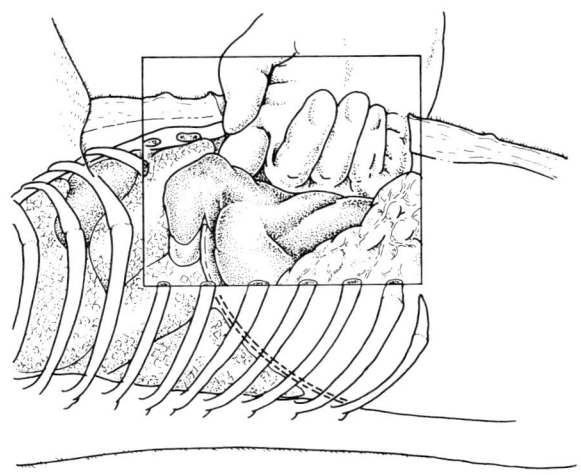

Fig. 3.19. The elevation of a trapped liver lobe.

Pulmonary lobectomy

Indications

Pulmonary neoplasia, bullous emphysema leading to persistent pneumothorax, torsion of a lung lobe, biopsy and infection of a lobe due to the presence of a foreign body.

Equipment

A routine surgical set, plus right-angled bronchial forceps (non-crushing), or a large curved haemostat, and gelatin foam (Gelfoam, Upjohn Ltd).

Technique

The thorax is opened on the left or right side at the fifth intercostal space. The lobe or lobes to be removed are identified and mobilized from the periphery inwards. If infection is suspected then packing off the remaining area with swabs may be carried out if space permits. The pulmonary vessels should be isolated and ligated twice, close to their origin and close to the lung lobe. The pulmonary vessels are relatively short and both veins and arteries are thin-walled. Gentle pressure with a moist swab will allow exposure of the vessels rather than the use of instruments.

Following the ligation and transection of the vessels between the ligatures the bronchus is then divided (Fig. 3.20a). An occluding clamp that does not crush the cartilaginous rings is preferable. An airtight seal of the bronchus is now required to avoid a pneumothorax. This is accomplished either by using a series of interrupted sutures laid so as to slightly invert the bronchial stump or a double layered continuous suture (Fig. 3.20b). Fine braided silk of 3-0 diameter on a fine curved needle is the easiest to use. Care should be taken in tensioning and tying the sutures not to tear the bronchial tissue beneath. This may be difficult to achieve where calcification of the bronchial rings is advanced. A small piece of gelatin foam or a patch of pericardium may be taken and sutured over the stump to aid sealing.

Following closure airtightness of the bronchus can be tested by flooding the area with saline, and following aspiration of fluid the chest may then be closed over the chest drain. The pleural dead space resulting will gradually become occupied by enlargement of the remaining lung lobes and vigorous re-inflation of lung lobes should *not* be carried out.

Partial lobectomy can also be carried out to remove small lesions or as a biopsy technique. The portion of the lung to be excised is separated over a crushing clamp; and the clamped area can then be kept sealed by oversewing with fine Dexon in a Cushing-type pattern. A small piece of Gelfoam can be held in place at the wound or a small piece of pleura or pericardium if a patch is required. However, such lung wounds will usually seal well provided they are not subjected to over-inflation by the anaesthetist.

Postoperative care

Routine antibiosis is required.

The chest drain should be attached to the chest bottle frequently as there is a danger of pneumothorax which because of the fragile nature of the mediastinum is life-threatening in the dog and cat.

Possible complications

Leakage of the bronchial stump, haemorrhage and pleural effusion are all possible complications of this procedure which may require a second exploration of the chest in the recalcitrant patient.

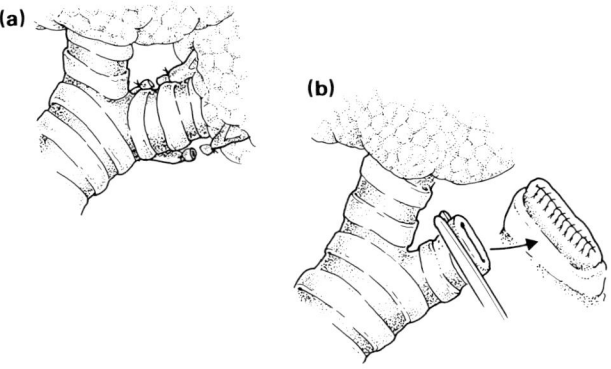

Fig. 3.20. The transection of a bronchus. (a) The blood vessels are ligatured and transected; (b) closure of the bronchus.

Chapter 4
Surgery of the Abdominal Alimentary Tract

HAROLD PEARSON

Ramstedt pyloromyotomy

Indications

The technique is used for the relief of pylorospasm or pyloric muscular hypertrophy, the facilitation of gastric emptying in cases of gastric dilation and torsion, and the removal of sub-mucosal pyloric polyps.

Equipment

A routine surgical set, plus fine-pointed straight Spencer–Wells haemostats and fine, straight, round-pointed Metzenbaum or equivalent scissors.

Technique

The pylorus lies near the roof of the peritoneal cavity on the right side of the abdomen, and is best approached through a midline laparotomy between the xiphisternum and the umbilicus. It is easily exposed by displacing the falciform fat and picking up the pyloric antrum of the stomach with Allis tissue forceps. The pylorus is suspended by a ligamentous fold of peritoneum which can usually be stretched to allow the pyloric canal and upper segment of the duodenum to be exteriorized, but in adult, deep-chested animals, it may be necessary to divide this attachment after double ligation of traversing blood vessels. The pyloric canal is then held tensed between finger and thumb with particular care not to touch the pancreas. A longitudinal incision varying in length, depending on the size of the animal, from 2.5–6 cm is made with a scalpel blade on the antimesenteric border of the pyloric canal extending for up to 1 cm along the duodenum, cutting through serosa only (Fig. 4.1). With the tissues still firmly tensed, the muscle layers, which may be of normal thickness or considerably hypertrophied, are gently divided until at one point the mucosa bulges through the incision as a noticeably separate layer of tissue with a pinker and somewhat glistening appearance. This manoeuvre is best performed by delicately scraping with the reverse side of the tip of the blade in order to avoid accidental perforation of the mucous membrane. Fine haemostats are then inserted with the jaws closed, almost parallel with the axis of the bowel, and by opening the jaws, mucosal and submucosal tissues are easily separated and the latter can then be cut with scissors. All visible strands of muscle tissue should be cut until the mucosa bulges freely along the length of the incision (Fig. 4.2). Particular care is needed in inserting the haemostats along the duodenum because at the junction of pylorus and intestine the tissues are less bulky and more tightly apposed. If the mucosa is inadvertently perforated it should be repaired immediately with fine absorbable sutures as soon as tissue separation has been established on either side of the perforation. Haemorrhage throughout is usually minimal with only scanty oozing from the sectioned muscle but bleeding points may be temporarily clamped or ligated. The bowel incision is not sutured. Multiple incisions have been recommended but one suffices and in very small puppies and kittens, only one is practicable. The operation is immediately effective and entirely safe although it may predispose to duodeno-gastric reflux. By contrast, alternative surgical procedures are not without risk. These are the Heinecke–Mickulicz and Finney pyloroplasties in which, respectively, the pyloric canal is incised longitudinally through all layers and then sutured transversely, and the pyloric antrum and descending duodenum are connected by a side-to-side anastomosis into a common stoma. The former procedure may seriously distort and narrow the pyloric lumen and the latter may occlude the adjacent bile duct.

Postoperative care

As the bowel lumen has not been opened, postoperative dietary restriction is not necessary. Recovery is usually rapid without complications.

Possible complications

None.

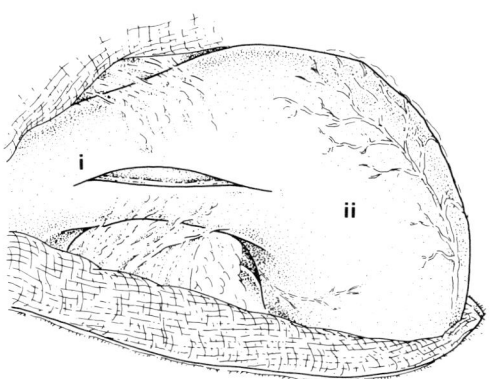

Fig. 4.1. Incision of the anti-mesenteric border of the pyloric canal. (i) The duodenum; (ii) the antrum of the stomach.

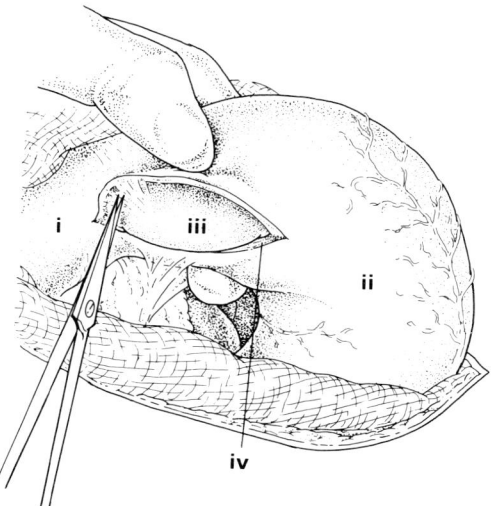

Fig. 4.2. Division of the muscle layers to expose the mucosa. (i) The duodenum; (ii) the antrum of the stomach; (iii) the pyloric mucosa; (iv) the pyloric musculature.

Partial gastrectomy

Indications

The technique is used in the treatment of fibrotic pyloric stenosis, multiple pyloric submucosal polyps, gastric carcinoma, bleeding or chronic fibrotic gastric ulcers, multiple gastric mucosal polyps, and fundic necrosis following acute gastric dilation/torsion.

Equipment

A routine surgical set, plus Lane intestinal forceps and Pozzi abdominal or malleable retractors, or equivalent instruments. A cutting diathermy facility is helpful but not essential.

For all operations in which the gut lumen is opened, sufficient equipment should be available to allow the laparotomy to be repaired with uncontaminated instruments and the hands should be immersed in antiseptic solution when bowel closure is complete.

Technique

The stomach is best approached through a midline laparotomy immediately behind the xiphisternum. The small intestines and spleen are displaced caudally and held out of the operation field by retractors.

The stomach is then palpated to assess the site and extent of the lesion which will probably affect either the fundus or the pyloric antrum. Lesions which require partial gastrectomy are usually readily palpable but preliminary exploratory gastrotomy may be necessary immediately adjacent to the mass or on the greater curvature of the fundus if no abnormality is palpable. In cases of possible malignancy the local lymph nodes should be carefully examined because surgery is not justified if metastases have occurred. In the absence of metastases it is often impossible to distinguish between malignant and benign ulcerative change without biopsy examination, but if this facility is not available, the decision whether or not to resect should be based on the assumption that in older dogs, carcinoma formation is more likely than chronic benign ulceration.

One of two techniques (Douglas *et al.* 1970) is likely to be appropriate:

1 In a minority of cases, a circumscribed lesion can be dealt with by local but liberal excision and simple suturing of the defect.

2 More frequently, the lesion lies on the pyloric antrum or pyloric canal and requires resection of this section of the stomach (Fig. 4.3a) and repair by direct gastro-duodenostomy (Figs 4.3b and 4.4) or closure of the duodenal stump and gastro-jejunostomy (Fig. 4.3c) or closure of both duodenal and gastric stumps, followed by a separate gastro-jejunostomy (Fig. 4.3d).

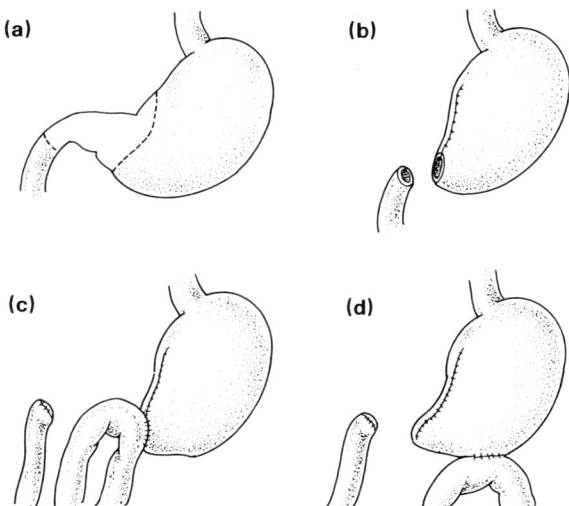

Fig. 4.3. Partial gastrectomy. (a) Before removal of diseased pyloric tissue; (b) repair by direct gastro-duodenostomy; (c) repair by closure of the duodenal stump and gastro-jejunostomy; (d) repair by closure of both the duodenal and gastric stumps, followed by a separate gastro-jejunostomy.

In limited excision of fundic lesions, the greater or lesser omentum may need to be divided after careful double ligation to control haemorrhage. Depending on the site of the lesion, it may then be helpful to isolate the lesion between two clamps. Diathermy division of the stomach results in less haemorrhage than sharp incision but large bleeding points still require ligation. The gastric defect is then easily repaired with two rows of continuous Lembert sutures of 2-0 or 3-0 Dexon or catgut. Resection of the pyloric part of the stomach is a less simple procedure and care is essential throughout to avoid damaging either the pancreas or common bile duct. The excision begins with division of the lesser omentum and meso-duodenum between ligatures close to the bowel. Two pairs of bowel clamps are then placed at least 1 cm apart on either side of the tissue to be resected and excision is performed with diathermy or scalpel, as close as possible to the inner pairs of forceps (Fig. 4.4a). Bleeding vessels in the meso-duodenum and divided stomach require immediate ligation. The method of restoring gastro-intestinal continuity should be carefully considered. It is technically easier to close the gastric and duodenal stumps and create a fresh stoma by gastro-jejunostomy but experience suggests that a stomal ulcer may well develop in the jejunum some time later. For this reason, direct anastomosis of the stomach to the duodenal stump is preferred despite the difference in stomal diameters. The repair is begun by closing the deeper (peritoneal) part of the gastric wound with a continuous Lembert suture until it is only slightly larger than the calibre of the duodenum (Fig. 4.4b). The anastomosis begins with stay Lembert sutures through the mesenteric and antimesenteric borders of the duodenum and apposed remodelled gastric stump. Tension by an assistant on these stitches not only stretches the stomata but also helps in elevating the duodenum for further suturing. Particular attention is paid to stitches at the attachment of the meso-duodenum which should be separated slightly to ensure adequate engagement of the bowel wall. The anastomosis is completed with interrupted Lembert sutures on the upper and lower edges of the bowel circumference between the stay sutures (Fig. 4.4c). Repair of the divided peritoneum is not usually necessary and the laparotomy is closed routinely.

Postoperative care

Pethidine analgesia is advisable for 24 h; parenteral antibiotic therapy may be maintained for 5 days but there is little risk of bacterial peritonitis because of the scanty intestinal flora at this level of the bowel. Intravenous fluid infusion is continued for 24 h during which time nothing is given by mouth. On the second day, oral fluids, preferably warm water or saline, are offered in 30-ml quantities every hour, followed by more substantial liquid food from the second day onwards. Solid food of light consistence is safe on the fourth day if fluids have not been vomited.

Possible complications

Blood-stained gastric fluid is usually vomited soon after recovery from anaesthesia. Postoperative ileus is uncommon after this operation but if vomiting continues, oral fluids are withheld and hydration is maintained with intravenous infusions.

Persistent vomiting may be due to breakdown of the anastomosis or iatrogenic pancreatitis but these complications are unlikely if the operation is performed properly.

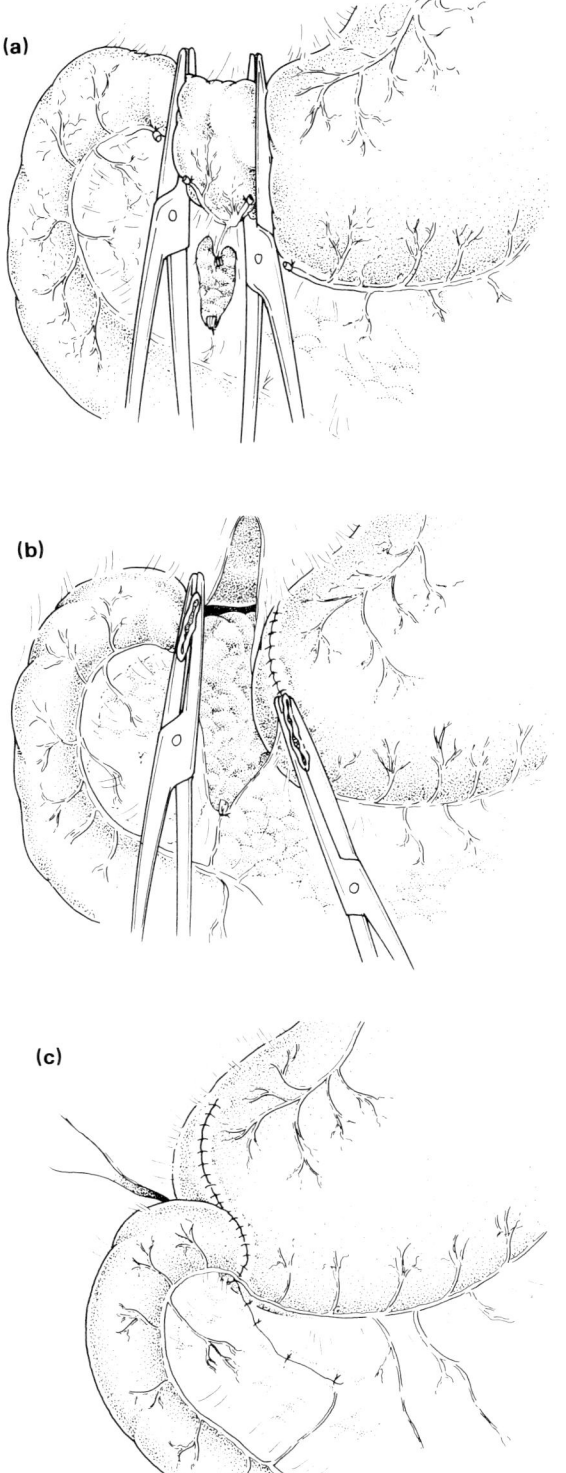

Fig. 4.4. Partial gastrectomy and repair by direct gastro-jejunostomy.
(a) Bowel clamps being used to isolate the tissue to be resected; (b) closure
of the deeper part of the gastric wound; (c) the completed gastro-
duodenostomy.

Gastrotomy, enterotomy, enterectomy and intestinal anastomosis

It is important to emphasize that animals with intestinal obstruction may be severely dehydrated and it is prudent in many cases to delay surgery for the removal of an intestinal foreign body or reduction of an intussusception until circulatory status has been restored by adequate infusion of intravenous fluids over a period of up to 24 h if necessary. Such therapy may be more important than competent surgery in determining the outcome of the operation. In all animals undergoing intestinal surgery provision should be made for intravenous fluid infusion over a period of up to 2 or 3 days.

Equipment

A routine surgical set plus up to four bowel clamps. For all intestinal procedures sufficient instruments should be available to allow those used for intestinal surgery to be discarded before the laparotomy is repaired.

Gastrotomy

Indications

The technique is used in the removal of gastric foreign bodies which cannot be withdrawn up the oesophagus and which are unlikely to pass through the bowel without causing an obstruction, the exploration of the gastric mucosa for lesions which cannot be palpated through the stomach wall, and, occasionally, the removal of a foreign body from the thoracic oesophagus but this is not usually the technique of choice for oesophageal obstruction.

Technique

The stomach is best approached through a midline laparotomy between the xiphisternum and umbilicus. Gastrotomy is usually performed for the removal of foreign bodies which can be isolated with bowel forceps in a pouch of the stomach along its greater curvature. Repair is simple with two rows of continuous Lembert 2-0 or 3-0 absorbable sutures, there being no danger of excessive inversion in the stomach. Needles and fish hooks which sometimes have to be removed surgically can often be manipulated through the stomach wall without gastrotomy. Exploratory gastrotomy for the location of foreign bodies and pathological lesions not palpable through the stomach wall is best performed by first inserting the blades of two bowel clamps side by side through a stab incision in the greater curvature and then opening the lumen by diathermy or scalpel between the closed bowel forceps (Fig. 4.5). Using this procedure haemorrhage from the incision is minimal; in repair, the first row of Lembert sutures is placed over the forceps which are progressively removed as the suturing proceeds.

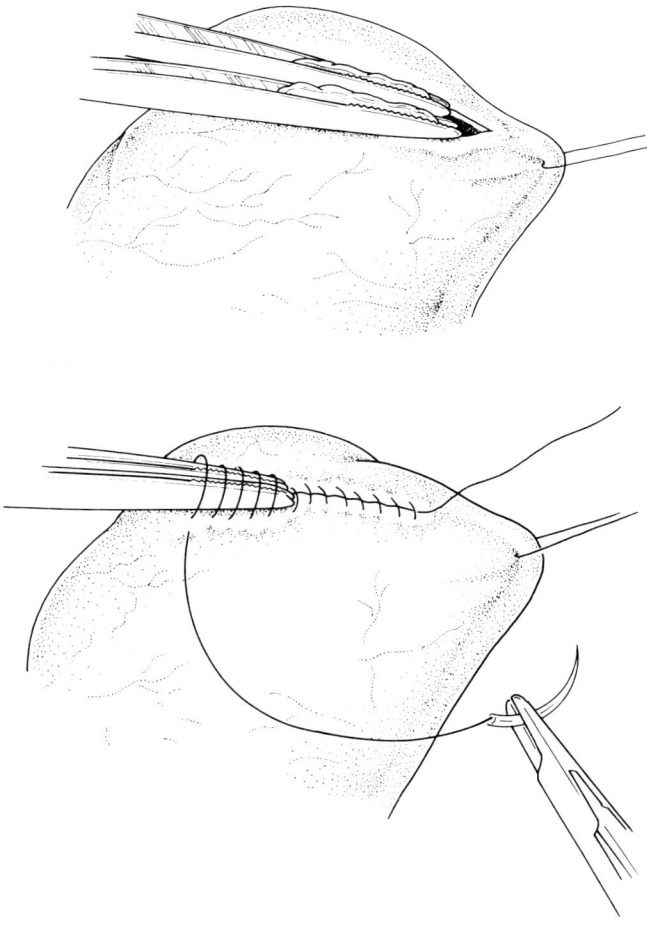

Fig. 4.5. Gastrotomy.

Enterotomy

Indications

The technique is used in the removal of intestinal foreign bodies which have not passed into the colon, and linear foreign bodies which may extend along the whole length of intestine, intestinal biopsy for histopathological diagnosis, to facilitate reduction of an intussusception which is otherwise irreducible and in occasional cases, to achieve intestinal decompression.

Technique

Enterotomy is best performed through a midline laparotomy centred on the umbilicus. The commonest indication is the removal of a foreign body which makes the obstructed segment of gut easily palpable for exteriorization. Throughout the operation, as little bowel as possible is exteriorized and this is bathed frequently with a sterile saline solution to prevent excessive drying. The fact that most foreign bodies are found in the jejunum or ileum suggests that peristalsis has a strong propulsive effect, but should a large or spiky object remain in one particular segment of bowel, pressure necrosis may rapidly develop making the gut vulnerable to rough handling. It is not uncommon in such cases for there to be multiple omental adhesions to the dilated loops of proximal intestine—such adhesions are reparative and should not be divided. Before the bowel is incised, the laparotomy is plugged with swabs to prevent peritoneal contamination with gut contents.

With any degree of bowel obstruction, the proximal gut is distended and bowel clamp or digital compression is essential to prevent leakage when the bowel is opened. It is usual also to apply clamps below the foreign body but this is not necessary if the distal gut is empty and contracted. Although it may seem advisable to incise healthy bowel on either side of the foreign body, it is usually easier to cut directly on to the object itself, making an incision long enough to prevent tearing during its removal. Care is taken to swab away bowel fluids which escape from the opened lumen. Most enterotomies can be repaired with little worry about bowel viability. Areas of severe pressure necrosis and discoloration should be observed carefully for several minutes if necessary for signs of revascularization and peristaltic movement before a decision is taken to resect. In bowel in which localized infarction is clearly present, usually on the antimesenteric border, the possibility of inverting such tissue with Lembert sutures through healthy gut should be considered as a safer alternative than resection. Enterotomy repair is effected using 2-0 or 3-0 absorbable material (Fig. 4.6). The best results are probably achieved with a single row of interrupted Lembert sutures but it is not essential to appose serosal surfaces (Fig. 4.6a). Gut of narrow calibre, as in small or immature animals, can safely be repaired with eversion sutures which least occlude the intestinal lumen. All sutures of whatever pattern must engage the submucosal tissue. When the clamp(s) is removed, gut contents can be squeezed past the suture line to test its integrity but with proper repair, this should not be necessary. After a final irrigation with saline, the segment of bowel should be wrapped in the omentum before replacement into the peritoneal cavity.

Linear or fabric foreign bodies may pose serious surgical problems in that they can extend from the stomach to the anus causing a plication or 'concertina' effect on the loops of small intestine which are tensed, sometimes to the point of multifocal perforation on the mesenteric border. In such cases it may be necessary to make a simultaneous gastrotomy and enterotomy to remove the bulk of the material from the stomach before teasing the remainder from the small intestine. The tightening and cutting effects of thin calibre materials of this sort, such as string or thread, can be so extreme that the material leaves the bowel lumen and lies entirely in the adjacent mesentery. Linear foreign bodies are best removed by tensing the material with haemostat forceps through an enterotomy midway along the affected bowel and then gently disengaging it from the distal and proximal loops. Multiple incisions are occasionally necessary. After repair of the gut, its mesenteric border should be carefully inspected for perforations which could leak and cause peritonitis. Small perforations might heal spontaneously, but all should be sutured. The affected loops of gut may be severely congested but they are seldom infarcted and resection is rarely necessary.

Enterotomy for biopsy purposes consists simply of a stab incision for removal of a sliver of bowel wall (which must include mucosa) at at least three sites, arbitrarily the duodenum, jejunum and ileum, in case the pathological change is confined to only certain segments of the gut.

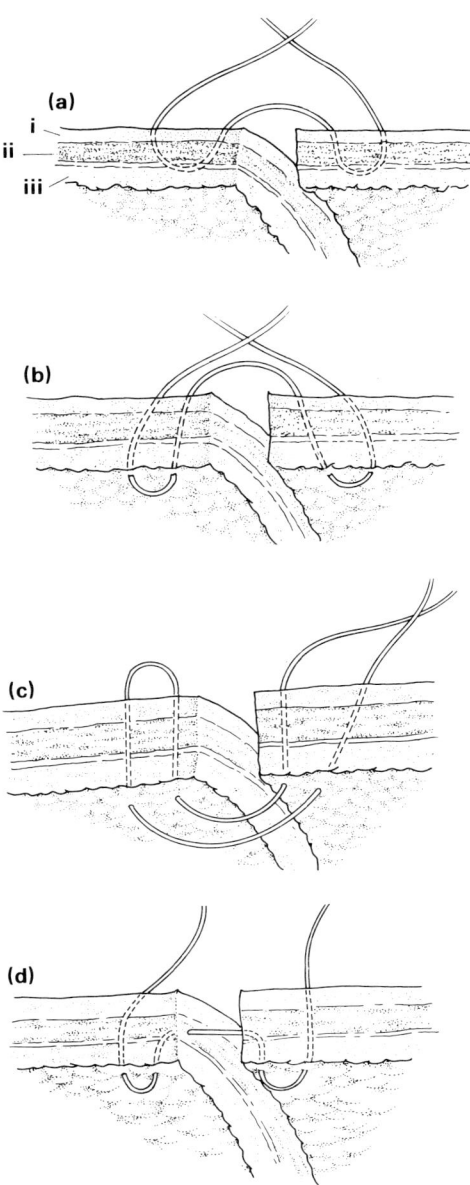

Fig. 4.6. Suture patterns for enterotomy repair. (a) The Lembert suture (inversion), (i) serosa; (ii) muscularis; (iii) mucosa. (b) Connell suture. (c) Eversion suture. (d) Gambee (crushing) suture

Enterectomy and intestinal anastomosis

Indications

The technique is used in the treatment of irreducible intussusception, primary circumscribed intestinal neoplasia, intestinal infarction especially after 'closed loop' obstruction or mesenteric stripping, severe intestinal trauma following foreign body obstruction or evisceration, obstructing intestinal adhesions, and intestinal stricture following, for example, previous surgery, sloughing of an intussusception (or localized polypoid change in cats).

The operation of gut resection and anastomosis is not without risk in unpractised hands and it should not be performed unnecessarily. The commonest indication is probably irreducible intussusception but such lesions can often be dealt with satisfactorily by enterotomy rather than enterectomy. In many cases of foreign body or closed loop obstruction, the need for resection depends entirely on whether or not the bowel is still viable. Gross infarction with gangrenous change is easily recognizable—the bowel is usually blackish-green in colour with no sign of peristalsis, noticeable thinning of its wall and a rapidly drying and glistening serosa. With less serious pathological change, the gut may be severely congested with intense blackish-purple discoloration but still remain viable—such bowel should be observed carefully, for several minutes if necessary, for signs of gradual venous drainage and arterial revascularization, although evidence of continued vascularity is not in itself a reliable index of viability especially after closed loop obstruction. A more dependable sign is the return of progressive peristaltic movement from adjacent gut towards the centre of the lesion. Similarly, after reduction of an intussusception, the affected segment of bowel may be so blanched in colour as to appear ischaemic with almost fibrous rigidity at the level of invagination but it remains viable and need not be resected.

Technique

Mention must be made of the classical Parker–Kerr method of resection and end-to-end anastomosis in which the intestinal loops remain closed throughout the procedure. Despite its apparent advantages, the method will often be found to be impracticable, especially in gut that is obstructed or in very young or small animals, and alternative methods are preferred.

Irrespective of how the anastomosis is to be performed, a standard technique of resection can be adopted (Fig. 4.7). With the affected segment of gut exteriorized, the laparotomy is sealed with swabs to prevent peritoneal contamination.

Intestinal contents are milked out of the gut, which is then isolated on both sides with two pairs of bowel clamps placed 2 cm apart, and its blood vessels are ligated individually in the mesentery. The bowel is then resected between the forceps, close to the inner pair, along with its mesentery. A common problem if end-to-end anastomosis is intended in cases of obstruction or if the ileo-colic valve is to be resected, is disparity in lumen size of the bowel stumps. This can be partially overcome by cutting the narrower segment of bowel obliquely, taking care to maintain vascularity by leaving more tissue on the mesenteric than on the antimesenteric border. After resection, bleeding vessels at the attachment of mesentery to bowel should be ligated and gut contents leaking from the stumps are swabbed away. For clinical purposes, most anastomoses are perfomed in one of three ways:

1 end-to-end (Fig. 4.8a),
2 side-to-side (Fig. 4.8b),
3 telescoping (Fig. 4.8c).

In recent years, the telescoping or 'sutureless' method (Fig. 4.8c) of drawing one stump into the other has been assessed experimentally in several species with good results, but the obvious difficulty in drawing dilated proximal bowel into contracted distal bowel would seem to make it impracticable for clinical anastomoses.

By contrast, the side-to-side method (Fig. 4.8b) has the advantage of allowing stumps of disparate size to be anastomosed with a stoma of adequate calibre and two rows of sutures to strengthen the anastomosis. The technique is widely used in practice but it has two particular disadvantages. Firstly, it inevitably distorts the bowel lumen and may predispose to stagnation of bowel contents, especially in the proximal blind stump. Secondly, with narrow bowel, it can result in considerable tension on the stoma, sometimes to the extent of occluding it.

For these reasons, simple end-to-end anastomosis (Fig. 4.8a) may be considered the technique of choice despite the difficulty of disparate lumen size. In bowel of adequate calibre, Lembert inversion sutures, in one row only, are satisfactory, but with narrow or immature gut as in cats or puppies, simple apposing or eversion sutures may be safer (Fig. 4.6 and Fig. 11 in Section 1). A continuous or interrupted suture can be used, but interrupted sutures have a less constrictive effect on the anastomosis.

The weak point in end-to-end anastomoses is the mesenteric border of bowel where improperly placed sutures may fail to engage the intestinal submucosa—slight separation of the mesentery will obviate this danger. The anastomosis begins with stay sutures on the mesenteric and antimesenteric edges of the apposed stumps. Troublesome everted mucosa can be excised but this should not be necessary if the stomata are stretched by tensing the stay sutures. Sutures of absorbable material are then placed carefully and not too tightly, preferably with a straight atraumatic swaged-on needle, around the circumference of the bowel, and the anastomosis is completed by repairing the mesenteric defect to prevent subsequent incarceration of loops of intestine. Before wrapping the repaired bowel in omentum, it is advisable to test the integrity of the anastomosis by squeezing bowel contents through it and watching

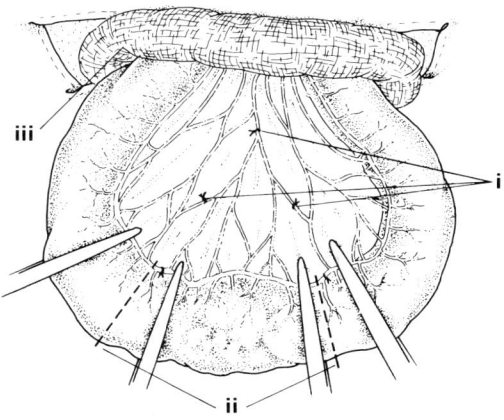

Fig. 4.7. Enterectomy. (i) Ligated blood vessels; (ii) lines of resection; (iii) laparotomy sealed with swabs.

carefully for leaks which might cause rapid fatal peritonitis.

Techniques are described for facilitating end-to-end anastomosis by approximating the enterectomy stumps for suturing over a bridging mould of material such as gelatin which subsequently dissolves, but this should not be necessary. In exceptional cases in which a considerable length of bowel is diseased, there may be concern about the possibility of secondary malabsorptive and metabolic effects of extensive resection. Published accounts of experimental resections suggest that 70–80% of the dog's small intestine can be removed without serious detriment, a proportion far in excess of what is generally necessary in clinical cases. Williams & Burrows (1981) have described the effect of short bowel syndrome after massive resection in a dog.

Whenever possible, the ileo-colic valve should be preserved primarily because of its functional value but also to avoid the difficulty of anastomosing ileum and colon. For these reasons an attempt should always be made to reduce a colonic intussusception at least through the ileo-colic valve. If the valve must be sacrificed, the associated lymph nodes should be left *in situ*, except for resection of a carcinoma high in the ascending colon.

Although the meso-colon is short, resection of the colon is a relatively simple procedure because this segment of gut has a tough wall and a wide diameter. It is, however, heavily infected and preoperative sterilization of the gut may be advisable. After most enterectomies, the laparotomy is closed routinely but if the peritoneal cavity is heavily contaminated, usually as a result of bowel rupture, liberal lavage is necessary with antibiotics in a saline solution before closure, and provision should be made for postoperative irrigation and drainage by inserting and suturing perforated tubing through two stab incisions 10 cm or so apart in the ventral abdominal wall.

Postoperative care

Analgesic therapy is indicated overnight and antibiotic therapy is advisable for 3 or 4 days to reduce the risk of peritonitis which may cause ileus. After 24 h, it is safe to offer tepid water or saline by mouth in small volumes every hour unless vomiting continues. During the next 2 days more substantial oral fluids are maintained, followed by solid food of light consistency as soon as defaecation has occurred.

Possible complications

The crucial prognostic sign after enterotomy or enterectomy is defaecation which indicates the return of normal peristalsis. Postoperative ileus is probably less common in the dog than, for example, in the horse and man, but it is nevertheless a potentially serious complication of enterectomy in this species. Most dogs defaecate within 24 h of intestinal surgery, often passing fluid and gas explosively after obstruction, but in occasional cases defaecation may be delayed for as long as 4 days. As a general rule, only fluids should be offered by mouth until defaecation occurs. If vomiting continues, even fluids are withheld and it is then vitally important to resume intravenous fluid therapy for as long as the ileus persists. Animals which continue to vomit after discontinuation of oral fluids give real cause for concern because of the possibility of anastomosis breakdown and consequent fulminant and rapidly fatal peritonitis. In such cases, the results of radiography and paracentesis are usually equivocal and the clinician may reluctantly but quite properly decide to re-open the laparotomy and inspect the anastomosis only to find local peritoneal adhesions which should be gently divided. Provided fluid therapy is maintained, these cases generally recover satisfactorily. If, by mischance, the anastomosis has failed, a fresh resection is advisable. Ileus, of course, predisposes to peritoneal adhesions and peritonitis causes ileus. Fluid and electrolyte disturbances, especially hypokalaemia, also predispose to ileus: there is therefore an overwhelming need for fluid therapy not just to reduce the likelihood of postoperative atony but also to counteract its effects. The duration and severity of postoperative ileus might be reduced by decompression of obstructed bowel at surgery, but this procedure increases the risk of contamination and peritonitis.

In the immediate postoperative period it is likely, especially in young animals, that oedema at the site of anastomosis also has an occlusive effect on lumen diameter, but this subsides fairly quickly.

Stricture formation occurring several weeks after enterectomy is usually due to excessive inversion during anastomosis and is particularly associated with the inappropriate use of Lembert sutures. Rarely, intussusception develops at the site of enterectomy, even in animals outside the normal age-risk group for this disorder.

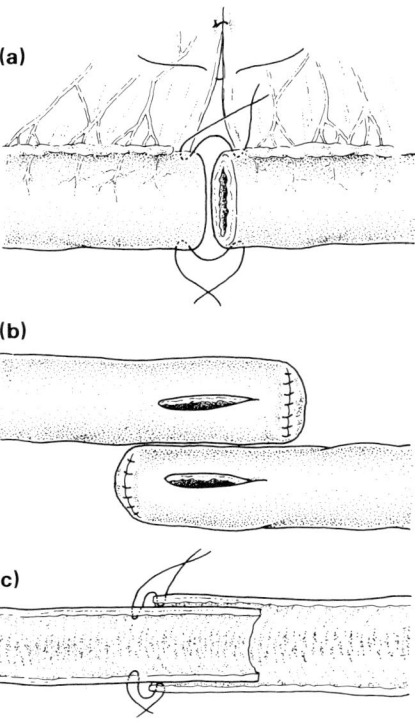

Fig. 4.8. Intestinal anastomosis. (a) End-to-end anastomosis; (b) side-to-side anastomosis; (c) telescoping anastomosis.

Intussusception surgery

Indications

As in children, intussusception in dogs is a juvenile disorder occurring mostly in animals less than 1 year of age. In these species, the lesion begins with invagination of jejunum into jejunum or jejunum into ileum, and as the intussusception lengthens the invaginated bowel passes through the ileo-colic valve and sometimes down the entire colon and through the anus. Regrettably, lesions which protrude from the anus are often misdiagnosed and treated for several days as rectal prolapses.

Equipment

A routine surgical set, plus four bowel clamps.

Techniques

In babies, more than 75% of intussusceptions can be reduced non-surgically by the hydrostatic pressure of a barium enema which is continued until multiple loops of small bowel are filled with contrast agent (Ravitch 1979). This technique is of value for the reduction of intussusceptions which develop in very young animals (of several species) during artificial rearing or at the time of premature weaning, provided that the lesion is diagnosed quickly. Warm saline solution is gently injected up the rectum and colon by means of a 60 cc syringe and narrow bore blunt-ended tube such as a 3 mm endotracheal tube, until the fluid no longer returns through the anus. In suitable cases, the method is surprisingly quick and simple.

Most intussusceptions are of longer duration and require surgical reduction. Non-surgical reduction by pressure on the apex of the invagination through the abdominal wall has been advocated, but the method carried unacceptable risks of bowel rupture and rapidly fatal peritonitis. Intussusceptions are usually easily exposed through a midline laparotomy but those which have prolapsed through the anus may first have to be repelled up the colon before they can be manipulated through the colon wall at the pelvic inlet. The correct method of reducing an intussusception is to milk it out with progressive finger and thumb pressure on its apex. Some lesions are quickly and easily reducible with no risk of bowel trauma. Others are totally irreducible because of adhesions which have developed between the serosal surfaces apposed by the invagination (Fig. 4.9). Paradoxically, the longer the intussusception the less likely is it that adhesions will have developed simply because the serosae are not in constant apposition during the progressive development of the invagination. Weaver (1977) found no relationship between the duration of signs, the length of the lesion or its reducibility.

In the dog, compound intussusceptions can occur; in such cases, the outer, more recent invagination is usually reducible, but the initial lesion may be firmly fixed by adhesions.

Irreducible intussusception is probably the commonest indication for enterectomy in the dog, but surgical procedures short of excision should first be attempted. It is always advisable and usually possible to reduce the lesion at least through the ileo-colic valve. Intussusception may prove irreducible because of either adhesions between apposed serosal surfaces or, more commonly, excessive tension on the outer rim of bowel possibly after most of the invagination has been reduced. Recent adhesions can sometimes be divided with haemostat forceps or scissors but the presence of firm solid adhesions is a clear indication for resection. Excessive tension on the outer layer of bowel is less serious and can usually be relieved quite safely. Forced reduction by apex pressure in lesions of this sort causes multiple, longitudinal sero-muscular tears on the outer rim of gut which may relieve the tension sufficiently for reduction to be completed. Such tears can extend haphazardly and it is preferable to relieve tension in a more controlled way by making longitudinal incisions down to the mucosa along the outer layer of bowel or alternatively, a single enterotomy which is subsequently sutured. Sero-muscular tears or incisions need not be repaired. After reduction of an intussusception, the site of invagination should be carefully examined for the presence of lesions such as linear foreign bodies or tissue masses which might predispose to recurrence. In reducible intussusceptions, the gut is usually viable although it may appear abnormally congested or ischaemic and feel diffusely fibrotic. In occasional cases, the intussusception may already have sloughed leaving a natural anastomosis and usually a clear fibrotic mesenteric scar, but the lumen is likely to be stenosed and resection is probably necessary because of chronic obstruction.

Postoperative care

Analgesia is advisable for 24 h to suppress any tendency to hyperperistalsis which can induce a rapidly fatal volvulus. The treatment otherwise is simply appropriate dietary restriction depending on whether or not the lumen has been opened, and careful observation for clinical signs of recurrence of the disorder.

Possible complications

The major complication is recurrence of the lesion either during the immediate postoperative period or at any time during the next few months. Ravitch (1979) quotes a recurrence rate of 4–5% in babies, and in Weaver's series of twenty-six dogs, five required further surgery within 20 days of the original operation, possibly because of predisposing enteric disease in these animals. The control of identifiable predisposing factors such as intercurrent

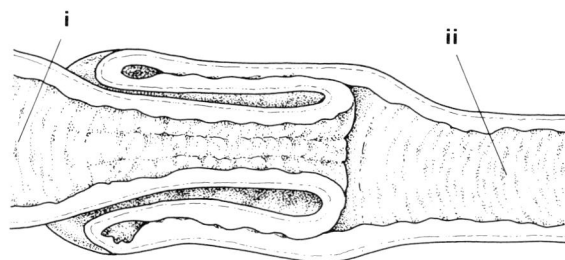

Fig. 4.9. Intussusception. (i) Proximal; (ii) distal.

intestinal parasitism or infection is therefore important particularly as lymphatic tissue enlargement in the terminal ileum is thought to be responsible for many human intussusceptions. Clinical experience suggests that the German Shepherd dog is most at risk for multiple recurrences. For recurrent cases, mesenteric plication or suturing mesentery diffusely to parietal peritoneum have been advocated as preventative techniques.

The treatment of gastric dilation and torsion

Indications

As above

Equipment

14–18 G gastrocentesis needles, a 16 mm outer diameter semirigid stomach tube, mouth gag and a 24–26 FR Foley catheter.

A routine surgical set will be required if gastrotomy or exploratory laparotomy are contemplated.

Techniques

The objectives, in order of urgency, in treating gastric dilation and torsion should be:

1 Immediate needle decompression of the stomach through the abdominal wall to relieve life-threatening tympany.

2 More effective non-invasive decompression by stomach tubing or temporary gastrostomy.

3 The institution of intensive intravenous supportive therapy.

4 Decompression by laparotomy if non-invasive methods fail.

5 Gastropexy by whatever method, and possibly pyloric surgery to facilitate gastric drainage as immediate or delayed preventive measures depending on which method of decompression has been used.

Gastrocentesis

The need for immediate palliative gastric decompression by needle puncture as a life-saving emergency procedure, by the owner if necessary, is not always appreciated. In animals suffering from acute respiratory and circulatory distress, a 14–18 G needle should immediately be inserted into the stomach through the abdominal wall, preferably in the lower right flank and if necessary at more than one site, to achieve partial relief of the tympany. Quicker decompression may be provided with a wide bore trocar and cannula but with a greatly increased risk of leakage from the stomach and consequent peritonitis.

This immediate crisis averted, the method of further decompression should be carefully considered. The conventional treatment of prompt laparotomy for evacuation of the stomach by gastrotomy is still widely practised, but there is now convincing evidence that other noninvasive methods result in a markedly better recovery rate and may, in fact, obviate the need for any surgical interference. Acute gastric dilation, even without volvulus, induces profound metabolic and circulatory disturbances which require supportive therapy before many patients are fit for abdominal surgery under general anaesthesia. Immediate laparotomy before a period of stabilization inflicts surgical trauma in an animal which may already be critically shocked with impending circulatory collapse. If this approach is still preferred despite these contraindications, it should be remembered that simultaneous fluid therapy is absolutely essential, but splenectomy, sometimes regarded as an integral part of the procedure, most certainly is not.

Alternative non-invasive techniques for gastric decompression were originally described by Funkquist & Garmer (1967) and Pass & Johnston (1973); more recent reports of modifications to each method (Funkquist & Obel 1979, Walshaw & Johnston 1976) are supported by improved recovery rates. The judicious use of these techniques permits effective decompression and stabilizing fluid therapy, without the need for immediate major surgery.

Decompression and aspiration of gastric contents by stomach tube

This technique aims at decompression by aspirating gastric contents through a stout stomach tube passed down the oesophagus with the animal fully conscious. An essential preliminary procedure is gastrocentesis with a long needle of 2 mm outer diameter inserted first through the lower right flank with the dog in the standing position and then at other sites on the right or left where tympany is most obvious on percussion. When the tympany has been sufficiently relieved for the abdomen to be reduced to normal size, a 16 mm outer diameter stomach tube of appropriate length is inserted through a wooden mouth gag and manipulated, preferably by fluoroscopy, through the cardia. The dog is then repeatedly rotated on its long axis until no further fluid can be aspirated. The less effective the preliminary needle decompression, the more difficulty is experienced in manipulating the tube into the stomach. After intubation and drainage through the tube, gastric lavage can then be performed through tubes of larger calibre. In case of difficulty in initial insertion, Funkquist & Obel (1979) describe a modified stomach tube fitted with a rigid extension guide to negotiate the constricted cardia. Dann (1976) recommends an essentially similar procedure, performed under light sedation, using a 14–16 G gastrocentesis needle and a slightly narrower stomach tube through which gastric contents are siphoned or aspirated into a glass reservoir jar by means of a small vacuum cleaner. A major advantage of this technique is that adequate decompression allows the stomach to return to its normal position without the need for immediate surgery, although Funkquist & Obel (1979) recommend radiographic monitoring of the position of the fundus continuously during the recovery period. Displacement of the fundus ventrally and to the right with elevation of the pylorus may persist for several days, but it is not considered serious unless further gas or food accumulation develops. Using this method, immediate laparotomy is indicated only

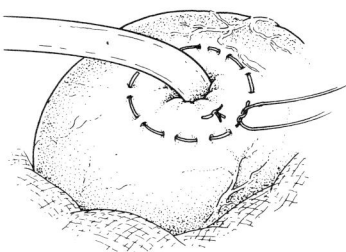

Fig. 4.10. Tube gastrostomy.

if decompression is inadequate or if fundic necrosis is suspected. Because of the high risk of recurrent dilation, Funkquist (1979) recommends routine laparotomy for prophylactic fundupexy 1–3 weeks after the acute episode.

Temporary gastrostomy

This method allows immediate direct gastric drainage through a gastrostomy performed·under local analgesia, again delaying major surgery until circulatory and metabolic crises have been averted by fluid supportive therapy. A more recent report of this technique (Walshaw & Johnston 1976) recommends initial needle decompression followed by attempted passage of a stomach tube for evacuation and gastric lavage. If intubation is impossible or causes serious additional stress, temporary gastrostomy is performed, usually without the need for sedation. The site is the most prominent point of distension in the right paracostal region. Under local analgesia, a 5 cm grid incision is made through the stretched abdominal wall 2 cm behind and parallel to the costal margin. The bulging stomach is then picked up, if necessary by first splitting the overlying omentum, with two stay sutures and its wall is stitched with a continuous suture directly to the edges of the skin wound. With the peritoneal cavity virtually sealed, the stomach is incised and its edges oversewn to control bleeding. Evacuation and lavage are then easily possible. After a period of stabilization, generally not exceeding 24 h, laparotomy is performed to excise the gastrostomy and repair the stomach wall, at the same time palpating the spleen and stomach for evidence of persisting torsion which necessitates a midline approach for repositioning and possibly splenectomy or excision of areas of fundic necrosis. In their protocol of treatment, Walshaw & Johnston (1976) do not recommend exploratory laparotomy if stomach tube or gastrostomy decompression has been effective unless such complications are suspected, but if the operation is necessary, tube gastrostomy is also performed.

Exploratory laparotomy

Exploratory midline laparotomy is indicated in gastric dilation or volvulus only if:
1 Alternative techniques of decompression have proved unsuccessful.

2 Persisting torsion of stomach or spleen, or fundic necrosis are suspected after decompression.
3 Prophylactic surgery to facilitate gastric emptying or some form of gastropexy is considered advisable.

Whatever the indication, the operation should be delayed whenever possible until fluid therapy has resulted in improvement of the animal's clinical status. If surgery is performed because of inability to achieve drainage by other means, it may still be possible to avoid gastrotomy by simultaneously rotating the stomach and manipulating a stomach tube through the cardia. The stomach is often opened in the mistaken belief that total evacuation is essential—in fact, peristalsis, when it returns, will take care of food debris which cannot be removed through a stomach tube or gastrostomy.

Similarly, there is no justification for routine splenectomy unless the organ is infarcted. If torsion persists, the spleen may be intensely swollen and congested, containing a considerable volume of blood which may be unnecessarily removed from the circulation by arbitrary splenectomy. Although it is inevitably displaced by gastric torsion, the spleen plays no part in the pathogenesis of the disorder. Ischaemic fundic necrosis is a well recognized complication of gastric dilation and volvulus, and may lead to spontaneous stomach rupture. Extensive partial gastrectomy is occasionally necessary (Dingwell & Eger 1976).

The significance of delayed gastric emptying as a factor predisposing to dilation is uncertain, but pyloromyotomy is probably a safe routine prophylactic procedure to improve gastric drainage, especially if the pylorus feels hypertrophied or in breeds such as the Boxer which are prone to pyloric dysfunction.

The other commonly performed prophylactic procedure is some form of gastropexy. Effective fixation of the stomach to parietal peritoneum may well protect against subsequent torsion but will not necessarily prevent simple dilation.

The conventional method of gastropexy by simply incorporating the stomach in the peritoneal layer of laparotomy closure is now largely discredited but alternative techniques have been described. A method recommended during laparotomy immediately after stabilization is tube gastrostomy (Parks & Greene 1976; Walshaw & Johnston 1976) in which a 24–26 FR Foley catheter is placed in the stomach through a stab wound in the right ventral abdomen 4 cm behind the last rib. The catheter is first drawn through several layers of the plicated greater omentum and then into the lumen of the gastric antrum between a pre-placed purse-string suture which is tied after inflation of the catheter bulb (Fig. 4.10). The stomach is drawn to parietal peritoneum by external traction on the catheter and anchored with silk sutures. Unless further gastric decompression is required during the recovery period, the tube is kept capped and is covered with a bandage to prevent dislodgement. It is removed after 5–7 days and the resultant fistula then closes by granulation.

Funkquist (1979), emphasizing the importance of fundic mobility in predisposing to torsion, recommends a different method of fundic gastropexy in which, up to 3 weeks after the acute episode, the fundus is first diffusely traumatized by thermo-cauterization or diathermy and then fixed by five or six rows of silk sutures to the medio-dorsal part of the left diaphragm and adjacent dorsal abdominal wall to the left of the aorta. Yet another technique for preventive gastropexy (Betts *et al.* 1976) incorporates the stomach wall in four separate layers of the abdominal wall during closure of a left paracostal laparotomy.

Postoperative care

Supportive fluid, antibiotic and possibly steroid therapy instituted at the outset of treatment should be continued until fluids can be taken safely again by mouth. In this disorder, more perhaps than in any other, facilities for monitoring blood gas, plasma electrolyte and fluid status are of the greatest value in determining appropriate treatment.

In general, nothing is offered by mouth until normal gastrointestinal peristalsis is resumed, and this is usually first manifested by loud borborygmi and faecal voiding. At the same time the animal becomes noticeably brighter and eager for fluids, which should be offered in small quantities frequently for a 36–48 h period with progressively more substantial fluid and light solid foods thereafter.

Possible complications

The major complication of successful surgery for acute gastric dilation and volvulus is recurrence of the disorder, often repeatedly until the animal eventually succumbs. For this reason, most authors advocate a combination of preventive surgical procedures as an integral part of operative relief, or at elective surgery later.

Definitive advice on prevention of the condition will depend on a clearer recognition of its direct and predisposing causes. Current concepts of its pathogenesis increasingly point to aerophagia as a principal cause and this probably could not be prevented. The advice otherwise must be to feed good quality food in small frequent meals with whatever additives might seem to be beneficial, to exercise susceptible stock sensibly, to monitor familial relationships of clinical cases, and most important of all, to train attendants to detect the earliest premonitory signs of tympany and how to relieve it as an emergency procedure by either needle gastrocentesis or gastric intubation.

Chapter 5
Surgery of the Urino-genital Tract

W. EDWARD ALLEN

Removal of the abdominal testes of cryptorchid dogs, and the abdominal gonads and tubular genitalia of intersexual dogs

Indications

In cryptorchid dogs, the removal of abdominal testes is advocated to prevent neoplasia. In intersexual dogs, such surgery prevents reproductive behaviour and phenomena associated with the gonads, and prevents further development of a phallus.

Equipment

A routine surgical set.

Technique

In male dogs and intersexual dogs with preputial development, make a caudal parapenile skin incision (Fig. 5.1). Bluntly dissect the subcutaneous facia and fat until the prominent branch of the recurrent superficial epigastric vein is located as it crosses the abdomen transversely towards the penis. Ligate and transect this vessel and apply haemostasis to other small vessels. Reflect the penis laterally. In intersexual dogs with no preputial development, make a midline caudal skin incision. Open into the abdominal cavity via the linea alba and incise back to the anterior brim of the pubis. Locate the urinary bladder and reflect this caudally. In cryptorchid dogs, the vasa deferentia can be easily identified as white, wire-like tubes diverging from the neck of the bladder. Gentle traction on each vas usually brings the small testicle with its rudimentary epididymis into view. On occasions the testis is in the inguinal canal, and the vas will disappear through the internal vaginal ring. Traction on the vas and pressure on the abdominal muscles at the external ring will replace the testis in the abdominal cavity. Both the vas and mesorchium are ligated and transected (Fig. 5.2).

In intersexual dogs, greater or lesser development of the Mullerian and/or mesonephric duct systems will have occurred and gonads will be ovaries, testes or ovotestes. The duct systems will be located, as in cryptorchid dogs, by caudal reflection of the bladder, and traction will bring the gonads into view. The gonads are freed by ligation and section of the mesurchium or mesovarium. Broad ligaments, if present, and the caudal genital tract are ligated and sectioned as for routine ovarohysterectomy, and the abdominal incision is closed in the normal way.

Postoperative care

Routine antibiosis. Prescrotal incisions for the routine removal of scrotal testes often cause irritation, and an Elizabethan collar should be fitted to prevent self-trauma.

Possible complications

Scrotal testes in cryptorchid dogs are usually obvious and should also be removed. In dogs which do not have two scrotal testes, and in intersexual dogs, the periscrotal and parapenile areas should be examined closely for the presence of descended but ectopic gonads, which can be very small. On occasion the testes lie subcutaneously on the medial aspect of the thigh. They can only be located by careful palpation after laparotomy has indicated that the vasa pass through the inguinal rings, but the testes cannot be pulled back into the abdomen.

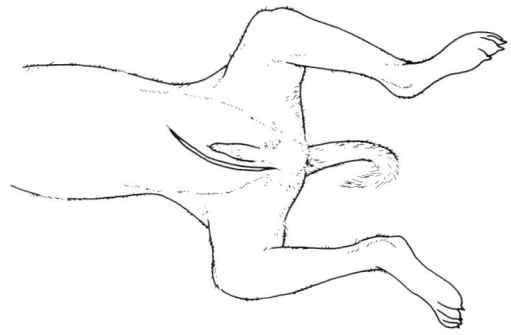

Fig. 5.1. The parapenile skin incision.

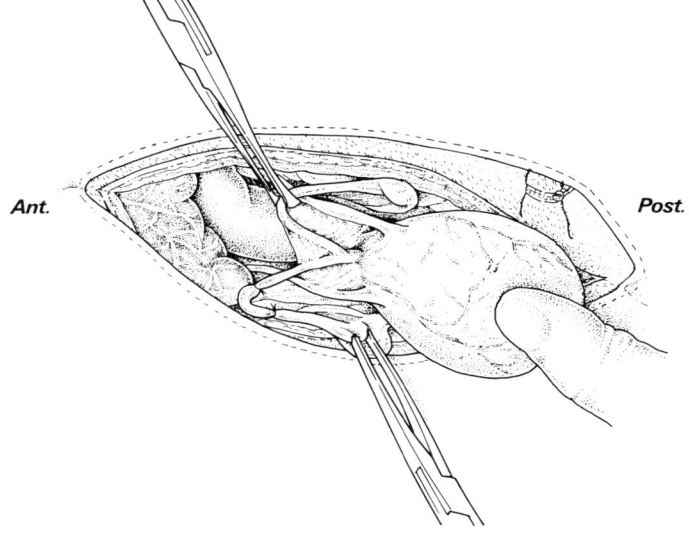

Fig. 5.2. Ligation and transection of the right vas deferens.

Episioplasty, episiotomy and vulvectomy to treat perivulvar dermatitis and necrotic vulvitis

Indication

Chronic dermatitis of perivulval skin folds, usually in fat bitches and associated with a small vulva. The condition may be exacerbated by urine scalding and self-trauma resulting in various degrees of necrosis of the vulval labia. The bitch is usually reluctant to allow local treatment.

Equipment

A routine surgical set, plus diathermy.

Technique

Place the bitch in ventral recumbancy with the hind quarters elevated, and plug the anus with cotton wool (Fig. 5.3). Tie the tail forward. After preparing and draping the site, make a midline episiotomy incision from the dorsal commisure of the vulva towards the anus, using the cautery blade. Deepen the incision through the underlying muscle until it enters the vagina. The extent to which perivulvar skin must be removed is now assessed and the skin incised (Fig. 5.4). The incision must be made in healthy skin. During positioning and preparation of the bitch, some of the perivulval folds may have become disturbed, but diseased skin is recognized either by evidence of an exudative dermatitis, or the presence of shiny cicatricial tissue. Diseased vulval labia are also best removed, as is also the clitoris if this is going to be left exposed following surgery. Retract the vulval lips with tissue forceps and incise with cautery along the muco-cutaneous junction of the vulva, to include all diseased tissue (Fig. 5.5). Dissect the area between the skin and vulval incisions free of the underlying subcutaneous tissue by blunt dissection. Large bleeding vessels should be dealt with as they are found, but capillary ooze is best left as this will stop when the wound is closed. After removal of all proposed skin (Fig. 5.6), the wound is closed by simple interrupted sutures with buried knots, using polyglycolic acid (Fig. 5.7). Any exposed vestibular mucosa at this stage everts when the bitch regains a more natural position.

Postoperative care

Routine antibiosis. An Elizabethan collar may have to be fitted to prevent self-trauma during healing, but irritation is usually minimal.

Possible complications

Due to the difficulty in assessing the amount of skin to be removed in order to ablate all the perivulvar folds, it may be necessary to re-operate at a later date.

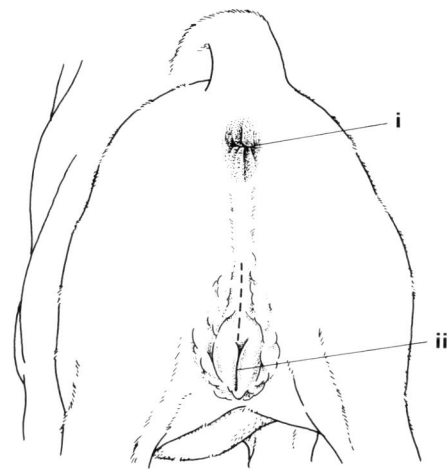

Fig. 5.3. Position for episioplasty, episiotomy and vulvectomy. The line of episiotomy is marked with dashes. (i) Anus; (ii) vulva.

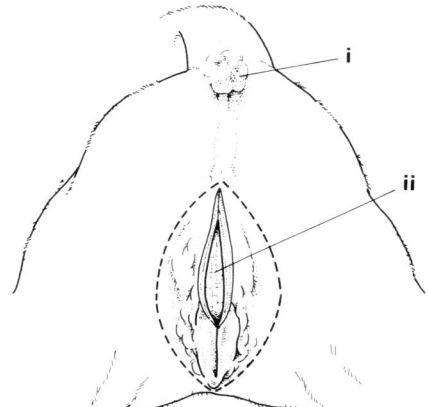

Fig. 5.4. Assessment of the perivulvar skin removal (dashes). (i) Anus plugged; (ii) the episiotomy incision.

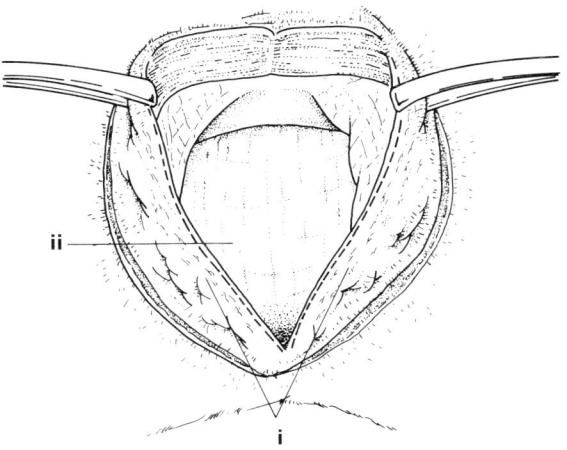

Fig. 5.5. Incision along the vulval muco-cutaneous junction (dashes). (i) Vulva; (ii) vesibule.

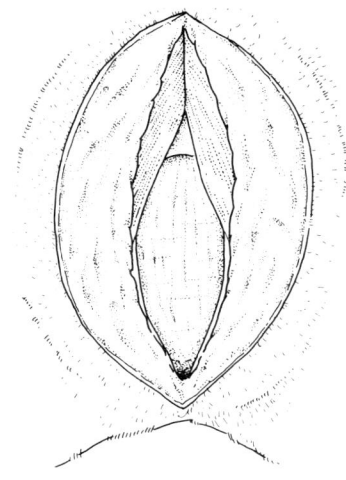

Fig. 5.6. The completed dissection including vulval tissue and the skin.

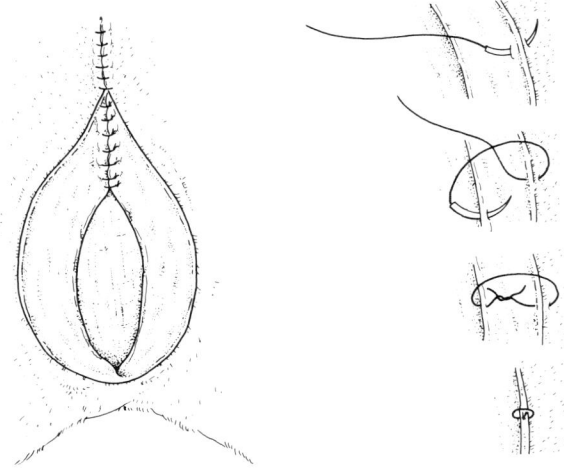

Fig. 5.7. Wound closure using a simple interrupted suture pattern.

Partial amputation of the penis

Indications

Traumatic injury, inability to retract the non-erect penis into the prepuce, and tumours. In intersexual dogs, the distal end of a protruding phallus can be removed in the same way. If hypospadia exists, it may not be necessary to involve the urethra.

Equipment

A routine surgical set, plus the appropriate sized male urethral catheter, bone forceps and a No. 11 scalpel blade.

Technique

Catheterize the urethra with the largest urinary catheter which can be passed comfortably. Reflect the prepuce and tightly tie on a 1 inch bandage proximal to the bulbus glandis. This acts as a tourniquet and is used to secure the penis vertically (Fig. 5.8). Make a stab incision into the midline of the dorsal surface of the penis and incise distally and laterally away from this point on both sides to produce a 'V'-shaped cut down to the os penis (Fig. 5.9). Repeat on the ventral surface, being careful not to incise the urethra which lies in the ventral groove of the os penis. Gently dissect the urethra off the os penis with a blade, keeping the cutting surface towards the bone. Free the urethra for about 1 cm distal to the base of incision and incise round its circumference at its distal attachment. Then cut the os penis as short as possible with bone forceps. Push the amputated distal portion of the penis along the catheter and out of the way (Fig. 5.10). The two sides of the 'V'-shaped flap are sutured together using 3-0 polyglycolic acid on an atraumatic needle. Simple interrupted sutures are closely apposed on either side of the urethra, which is still catheterized (Fig. 5.11). The urethra is then slit longitudinally with the blade, on a lateral surface, to its point of emergence from the penis, and sutured back flat over the stump (Fig. 5.12). The tourniquet is removed, and extra sutures placed at any points of haemorrhage. The dog is then castrated in the usual manner.

Postoperative care

Routine antibiosis.

Possible complications

Postoperative haemorrhage is rare, but if persistent the stump of the penis should be re-examined and resutured. Stricture of the urethra is also rare. If it occurs, further amputation or urethrostomy should be considered.

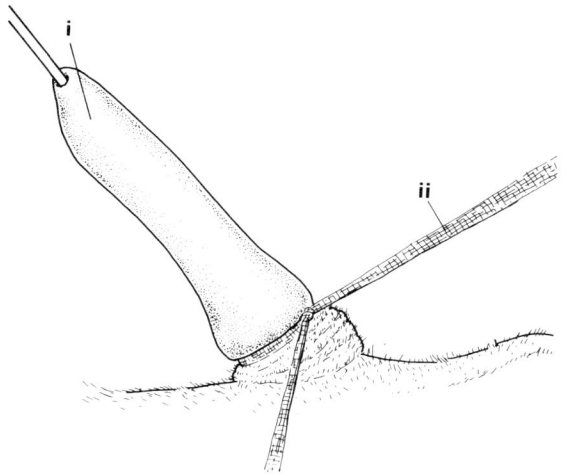

Fig. 5.8. Preparation of the penis. (i) Penis; (ii) the bandage tourniquet.

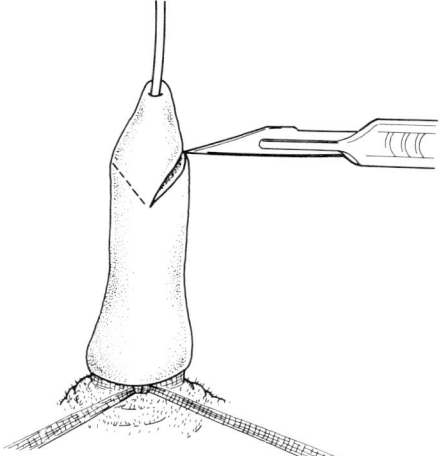

Fig. 5.9. V-shaped incision on the dorsal penis.

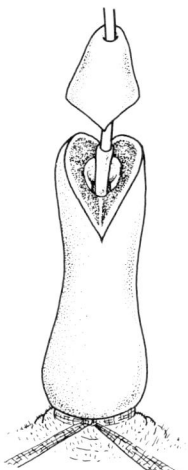

Fig. 5.10. Removal of the amputated portion.

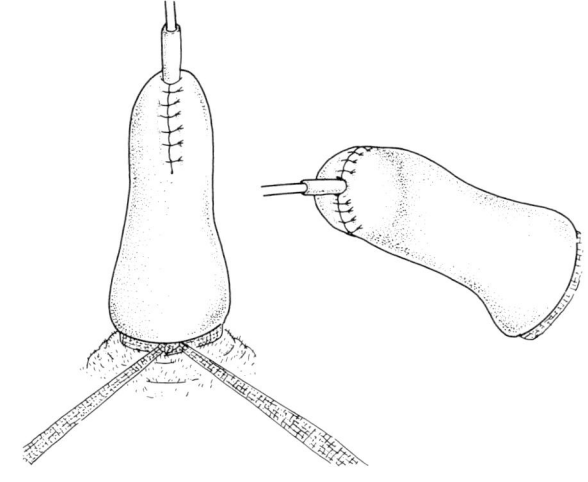

Fig. 5.11. Closure of the wound.

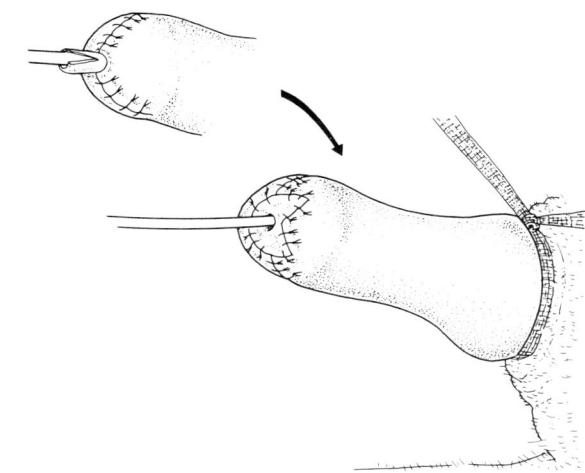

Fig. 5.12. Suturing the urethra back over the stump.

Removal of the prolapsed hyperplastic vagina

Indications

Complete vaginal prolapse (i.e. prolapse of the complete circumference of the vagina) is rare in the bitch. More commonly the ventral wall of the vagina, which becomes hyperplastic and oedematous during oestrus, is seen protruding from between the vulval lips (Fig. 5.13). The condition corrects itself after oestrus, but recurs at subsequent heats. Ovarohysterectomy is the treatment of choice in non-breeding bitches. In bitches required for breeding, the excess hyperplastic tissue must be removed, during oestrus, to prevent trauma and to allow normal coitus. The bitch can be mated at the next heat.

Equipment

A routine surgical set plus diathermy and a urinary catheter.

Technique

Perform an episiotomy, using the diathermy blade, as previously described. Continue the incision dorsally, sufficient to expose the whole of the hyperplastic vagina (Fig. 5.14). This is usually well circumscribed. Lift the hyperplastic mass, locate the urethral opening, and catheterize the urinary bladder (Fig. 5.14). Fix the catheter to the drapes with tissue forceps to prevent unintentional withdrawal. Retract the edges of the episiotomy incision dorsally with tissue forceps which can be anchored to the drapes using haemostats. Lift the mass and make a horizontal incision through the mucous membrane (but not through the submucosa) using the cautery blade, 1 cm dorsal to the urethral opening. Continue the incisions laterally and upwards on either side of the mass to meet dorsally. Now, starting dorsally, separate the mucosa from the submucosa using diathermy. This junction is best visualized as a gelatinous (oedematous) layer under the more solid mucosa. Manipulation of the mass is necessary in order to incise the mucosa at the depths of rugae. Do not attempt to stop capillary ooze at this stage, but continue to peel the hyperplastic mucosa downwards as it is separated, until the flap can be removed (the ventral limit of the excised tissue has already been marked) (Fig. 5.15). After removal of the mucosa, the submucosa tends to contract and reduce haemorrhage. Absorbable sutures with buried knots are placed transversely starting at the dorsal limit of the incision (Fig. 5.16). Following closure of the ventral vaginal mucosa, the mucosa of the episiotomy wound is sutured using absorbable material and starting dorsally. The knots lie under the mucosa, i.e. no knots protrude into the vaginal lumen (Fig. 5.17). If the dorsal vaginal wall and perineum are oedematous, a continuous suture may be necessary to eliminate dead space. Then close the perineal skin with interrupted sutures with buried knots, and remove the urinary catheter (Fig. 5.18).

Postoperative care

Routine antibiosis. An Elizabethan collar may have to be fitted to prevent self-trauma during healing, but irritation is usually minimal.

Possible complications

Rarely occur. Scar tissue formation in the vagina rarely interferes with subsequent mating or whelping.

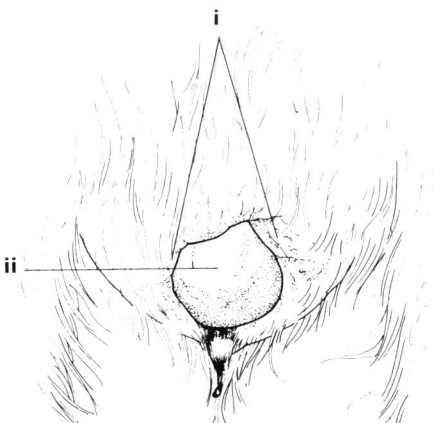

Fig. 5.13. The prolapsed hyperplastic vagina. (i) Swollen vulval lips; (ii) hyperplastic vaginal tissue.

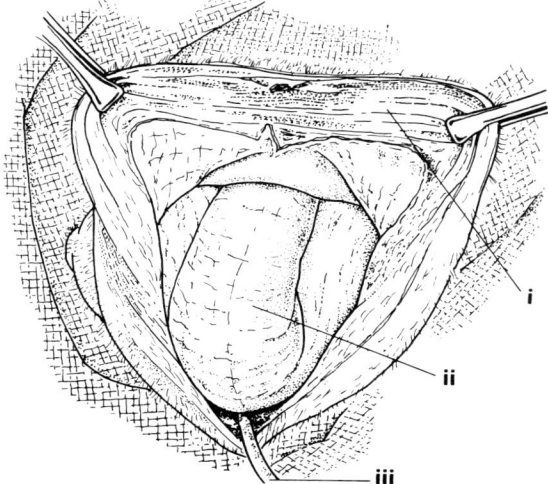

Fig. 5.14. The episiotomy wound to expose the vagina. (i) Episiotomy wound; (ii) vagina; (iii) catheter.

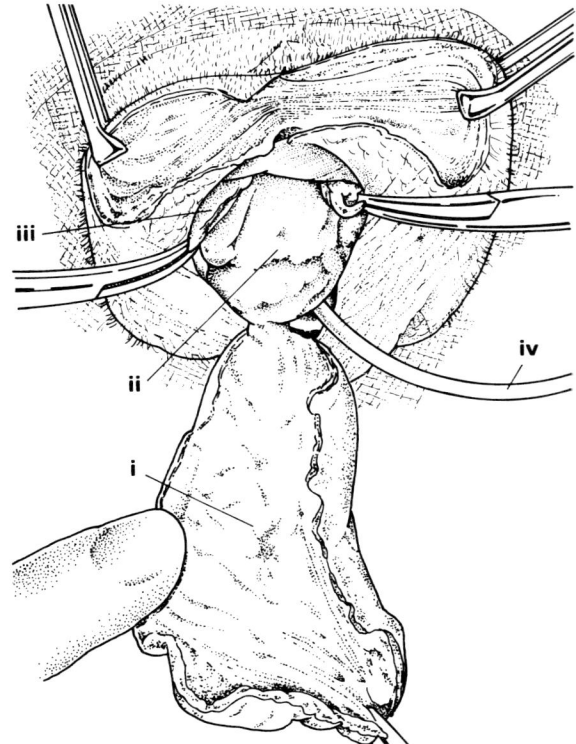

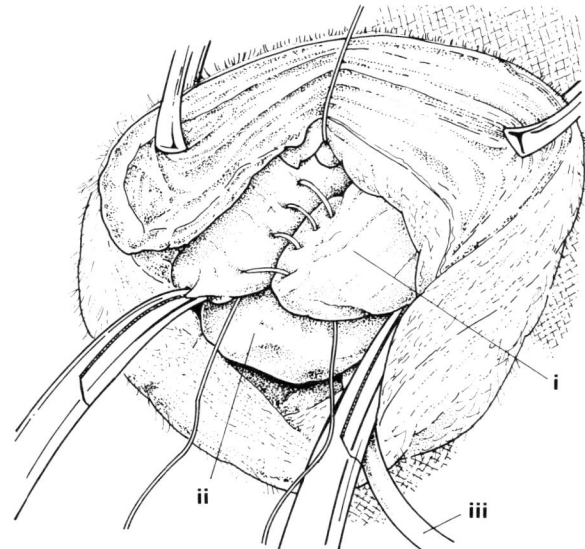

Fig. 5.16. Closure of the vaginal mucosa using a simple interrupted suture pattern. (i) Remaining vaginal mucosa coapted; (ii) exposed submucosa; (iii) catheter.

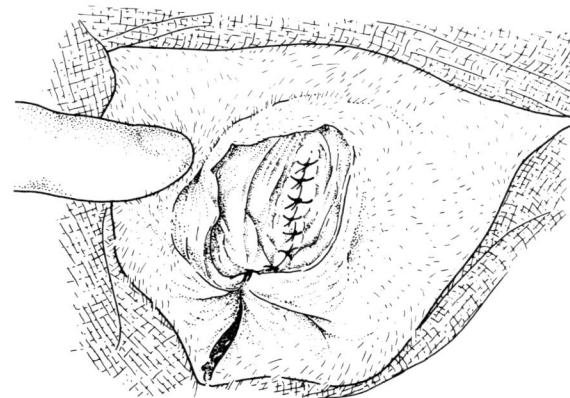

Fig. 5.17. The vaginal wound has been closed.

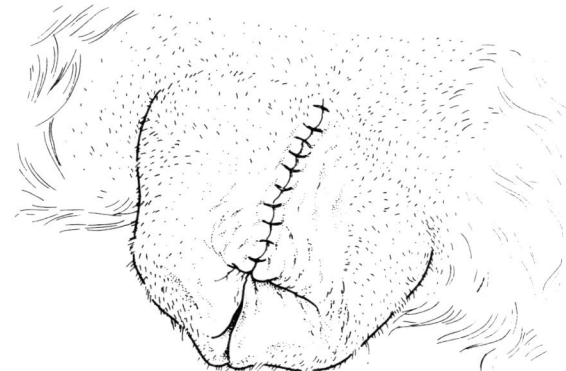

Fig. 5.18. Closure of the episiotomy wound.

Fig. 5.15. Removal of the hyperplastic mucosa. (i) Flap of mucosa; (ii) exposed submucosa; (iii) remaining vaginal mucosa; (iv) catheter.

Surgery to correct phimosis and paraphimosis

Indications

Phimosis

Inability to protrude the penis through the preputial orifice. Occasionally seen in puppies, where the preputial orifice can be minute. The dog urinates into the preputial cavity and urine subsequently escapes slowly through the orifice. There may be some separation of preputial skin from the mucous membrane lining the sheath, due to under-running with urine. The preputial opening must be enlarged.

Paraphimosis

Inability to retract the penis after it has been protruded through the preputial opening. This causes swelling of the exposed glans penis; it can usually be returned to the preputial cavity with the aid of lubricants, although general anaesthesia may be necessary. The preputial orifice subsequently needs enlarging.

Equipment

A routine surgical set.

Technique

Place the dog in dorsal recumbancy. Clip the hair from the distal prepuce. If the penis can be exposed, remove any secretions from its surface with moist swabs. Do not allow disinfectants or spirit to enter the preputial cavity during surgical preparation of the prepuce. Insert the blunt tip of a pair of straight scissors into the preputial orifice, whilst stretching the prepuce forwards. Cut caudally in the ventral midline for about 1 cm (Fig. 5.19). The extent to which the orifice needs opening depends on its original size, and the size of the dog, but should be sufficient to allow free protrusion of the penis. If there is extensive separation of the skin from the mucosa, the dead space should be ablated with fine absorbable sutures (continuous). The edges of the cut mucosa and skin are coapted on each side with simple interrupted sutures with buried knots using a fine absorbable material (Fig. 5.20).

Postoperative care

Routine antibiosis. An Elizabethan collar may have to be fitted to the dog to prevent self-trauma to the wound during healing.

Possible complications

Excessive enlargement of the preputial orifice causes drying of the tip of the penis, irritation and self-trauma.

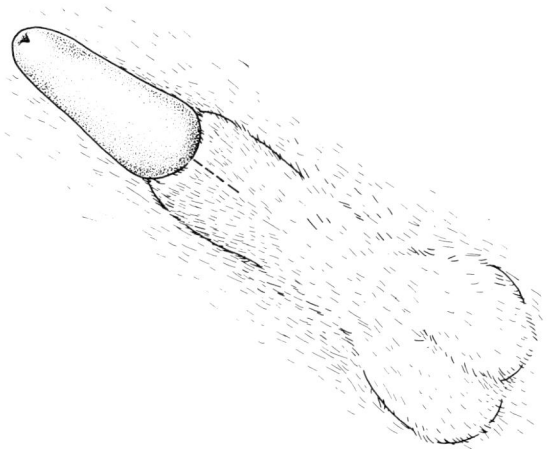

Fig. 5.19. Paraphimosis. The dashes mark the line of preputial incision.

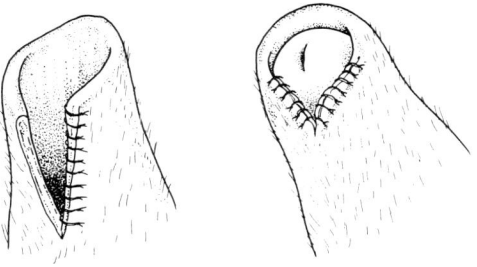

Fig. 5.20. Repair of the preputial wound.

Chapter 6
Ocular Surgery

KEITH C. BARNETT, PETER G. C. BEDFORD and
TERENCE D. GRIMES

Entropion surgery

Indications

Anatomical deformity of the eyelids involving an inward rolling of the lid margin resulting in conjunctivitis, keratitis, ulceration and epiphora (breed predisposition: Golden Retriever, Labrador Retriever). Compression of the lacrimal puncta and obliteration of the lacrimal lake (breed predisposition: Miniature Poodle, Toy Poodle). Conformational underdevelopment of the palpebral aperture (breed predisposition: Kerry Blue Terrier, Chow Chow). Conformational enophthalmos (breed predisposition: Dobermann Pinscher, Great Dane). Enopthalmos associated with phthisis bulbi.

Equipment

Scalpel with No. 11 and No. 15 disposable blades. A lid support in the form of an entropion clamp, a metal tongue depressor or spatula, needle holder. Fine smooth and rat-tooth forceps. Fine blunt and sharp pointed scissors. Small curved-on-straight 3/8 and 1/2 curved cutting needles. Fine silk, catgut and non-absorbable suture materials. Measuring calipers and ruler.

Techniques

The situation and extent of the lid deformity is assessed very carefully prior to the induction of general anaesthesia (Fig. 6.1). The defect is to be corrected by the removal of a strip of skin and orbicularis oculi muscle that is tailored to the required width and length so that as the wound is closed the normal conformation of the lid is restored.

Hair is close-clipped from the surgical site which is prepared with Betadine solution.

1 A lid support is introduced into the conjunctival sac and raised beneath the site of lid incision providing a firm base for exact and perpendicular section of the lid skin while haemorrhage is usefully controlled. This support may be provided by the surgeon's index finger.

A first incision is made parallel to the lid margin and 2–3 mm from it. A second delineates a strip of skin that is adjusted in width to the situation and severity of the entropion.

The strip is raised at one end and removal of the skin and underlying muscle is completed with fine pointed scissors (Fig. 6.2). Care is taken not to damage the deeper lying tarsal plate and conjunctiva. The skin wound only is closed using simple interrupted sutures of 3-0 Supramid (B. Braun Melsungen, W. Germany) or fine braided nylon. The suture ends are directed away from the lid edge (Fig. 6.3).

2 Correction of entropion involving both upper and lower lids at the lateral canthus (Fig. 6.4) is achieved by the removal of an angulated strip of skin and orbicularis muscle in the shape of an arrowhead adjacent to the lateral canthus.

The lid support is introduced into the conjunctival sac below the lateral canthus. Two incisions are made through the lid skin 3 mm from the lid edge and meeting at the canthus. A further pair of incisions meeting at a more acute angle delineate an arrowhead the length of which is related to the degree of inturning at the canthus. This skin is raised and removed with sharp scissors together with a superficial strip of the underlying orbicularis muscle (Fig. 6.5).

The first suture is laid so as to draw the residual margin of skin at the lateral canthus to the point of the arrow (Fig. 6.6). Further simple interrupted sutures of 3-0 Supramid complete the closure (Fig. 6.7).

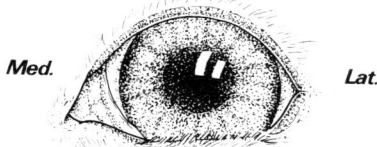

Fig. 6.1. Entropion, lower lid, left eye.

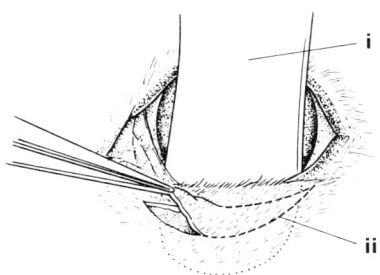

Fig. 6.2. Removal of the strips of skin and muscle. (i) Lid support; (ii) incision.

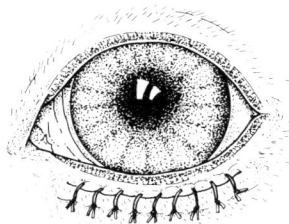

Fig. 6.3. Skin wound repair completed.

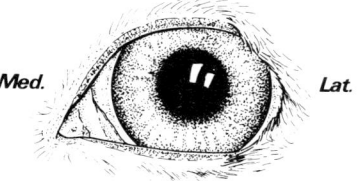

Fig. 6.4. Entropion involving both the upper and lower lids at the lateral canthus, left eye.

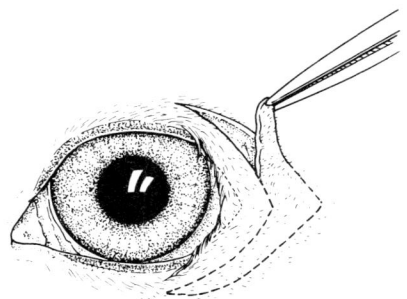

Fig. 6.5. The arrowhead of skin and muscle being removed.

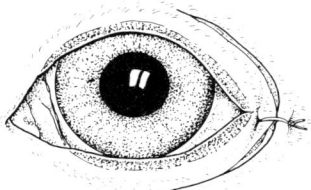

Fig. 6.6. The initial suture in the repair of the skin wound.

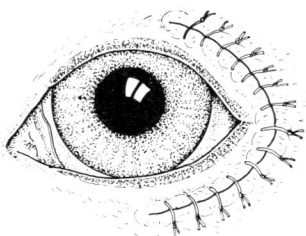

Fig. 6.7. Skin wound repair completed.

3 Correction of entropion involving upper and lower lids at the lateral canthus with ectropion of the lower lid. It is found that the lateral canthus is abnormally mobile and medially displaced upon the cornea.

The procedure again involves the removal of an arrowhead of skin adjacent to the lateral canthus (Fig. 6.8). However, the edges of the incision are undermined by blunt dissection and raised to permit identification of a wide band of orbicularis muscle fibres curving around the lateral canthus (Fig. 6.9) and also the palpation of the posterior margin of the orbital rim. A 2-0 suture of monofilament nylon is laid vertically and as deeply as possible into the orbicularis muscle and carried in a mattress pattern into the lateral periosteal structures of the zyomatic process of the temporal bone (Fig. 6.10). The tension of the suture is adjusted so as to bring the lateral canthus to a normal position before it is tied. During closure the skin edges are trimmed so that any residual entropion is abolished as the skin sutures are tied (Fig. 6.11).

Postoperative care

Immediately after surgery the eyelids and skin wounds are cleaned with moist cotton wool and then anointed daily with a steroid/antibiotic eye ointment. Sutures are removed after 10 days. If there is any tendency to wound interference a plastic bucket or Elizabethan collar is employed.

Possible complications

Overcorrection and undercorrection of the presenting condition are the major complications. The surgical aim should be towards undercorrection as reoperation involves only the removal of further tissue rather than a procedure to relieve induced ectropion. The fibrosis of wound healing will inevitably provide a greater degree of correction than exists at the completion of the operation.

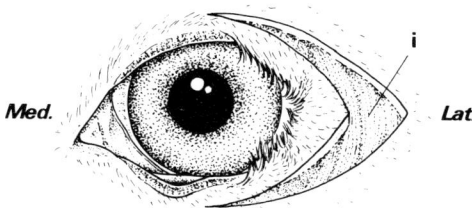

Fig. 6.8. The arrowhead skin resection (left eye). (i) Orbiculars oculi muscle.

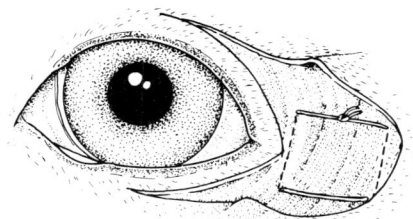

Fig. 6.10. The mattress tension suture.

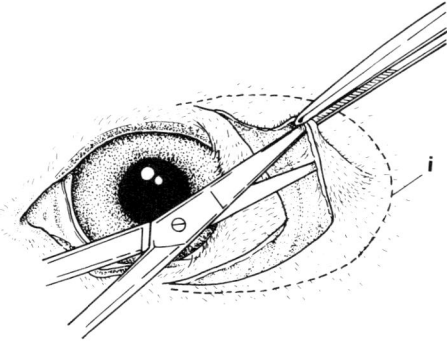

Fig. 6.9. Undermining the skin. (i) The extent of the blunt dissection.

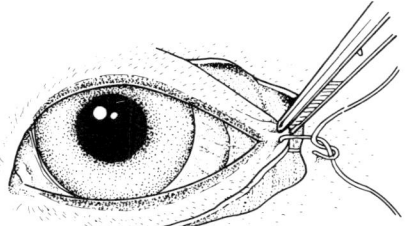

Fig. 6.11. Closure of the skin wound.

Ectropion surgery

Indications

Developmental deformity of the lower eyelid in which the lid hangs outwards and downwards away from the globe (Breed predisposition: Bassett Hound, Bulldog, Cocker Spaniel, English Springer Spaniel). Cicatrization with contracture following lid injury. Developmental oversize of the palpebral aperture. Paralysis of the orbicularis oculi muscle.

Equipment

As for entropion.

Techniques

1 Correction of cicatricial ectropion. Under general anaesthesia, the cicatrix is palpated and its depth and extent determined. A V-shaped incision is made through the lower lid skin and orbicularis muscle so that all scar tissue is contained beneath a ventrally directed flap (Fig. 6.12). The skin edges are undermined by sharp and blunt dissection. All scar tissue is removed and adhesions between skin muscle and fascia are released so that the tissue layers are normally mobile (Fig. 6.13). The deformed lid edge is raised to a normal position in relation to the globe, the V-shaped flap being pushed dorsally to accomplish this. The new position of the flap is rendered permanent by suturing the edges of the skin wound to form a Y-shape using 3-0 Supramid (Fig. 6.14).

2 Correction of ectropion by shortening of the lower lid combined with a supporting skin flap. Prior to general anaesthesia, the lid edges are inspected and a firm decision reached on the length of lower lid resection that is required to produce desired lid conformation (Fig. 6.15). A ruler or calipers may be used. The lower eyelid is split vertically into its skin/muscle and tarso/conjunctival layers to a depth of 1.5–2 cm. The lid is entered with a No. 11 disposable blade along the line of the Meibomian gland orifices as it is maintained in longitudinal tension between thumb and forefinger (Fig. 6.16).

The line of incision is continued beyond the lateral canthus, and following the upward curvature of the lower lid for a distance of 1–2 cm, the end point being determined by the degree of entropion that exists. A second incision is made from this point passing ventrally and slightly anteriorly ending at the horizontal level to which the lower lid has been split (Fig. 6.17). A continuous strip of lower lid skin and muscle and facial skin can now be dissected free and raised to expose the tarso/conjunctival layer.

A wedge of tarso/conjunctiva is removed from the lid to a marginal length that had already been decided (Fig. 6.18). The wedge is taken between the lid centre and the lateral canthus, but if the tarsal plate is buckled or distorted then this abnormal area is chosen for removal. The defect is repaired with interrupted sutures of 6-0 gut, the knots being placed on the subconjunctival surface (Fig. 6.19).

The skin flap is now drawn across the bed from which it was raised and a triangular piece of its lateral edge trimmed away (Fig. 6.20) so that when sutures of 3-0 Supramid are placed a suitable tension is given to the lower lid. The split lid margin is carefully coapted with interrupted 6-0 silk sutures which pass over the lid edges (Fig. 6.21). They are placed with moderate tension and knots facing away from the cornea.

Postoperative care

The lid edges are cleaned and treated daily with an antibiotic/steroid eye ointment. Any tendency to self-inflicted trauma is an indication for the use of a plastic bucket or Elizabethan collar. All sutures are removed in 10 days.

Possible complications

These include under- and overcorrection which should be avoided by careful measurement of the tissue to be removed. The lid margins heal well following splitting procedures if they are carefully reapposed. The loss of Meibomian secretion resulting from glandular damage appears to cause no problem.

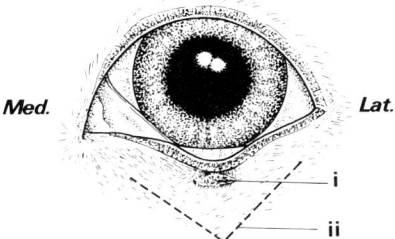

Fig. 6.12. Ectropion, lower lid, left eye. (i) The cicatrix; (ii) the line of incision.

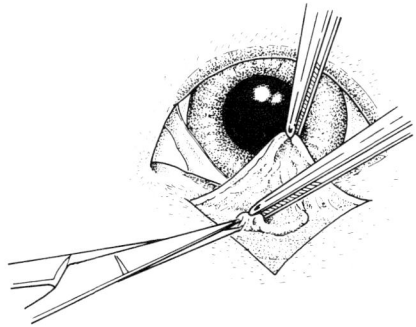

Fig. 6.13. Dissection of the cicatrix.

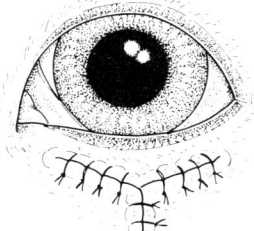

Fig. 6.14. The skin wound repaired as a Y.

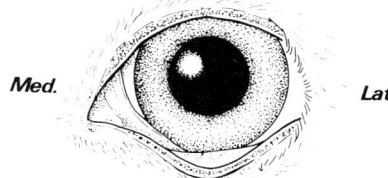

Fig. 6.15. Combined entropion and ectropion, left eye.

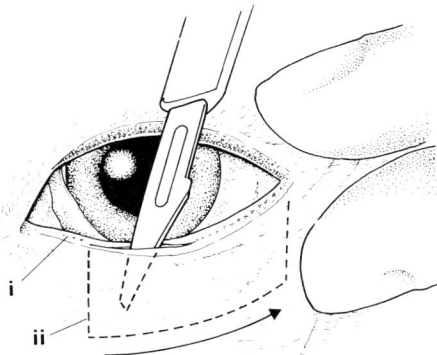

Fig. 6.16. The lid split. (i) Meibomian gland orifices; (ii) extent of undermining.

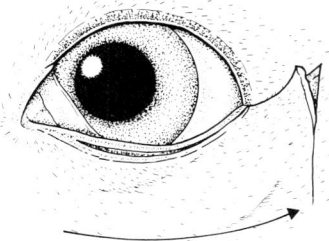

Fig. 6.17. Dissection of the skin flap.

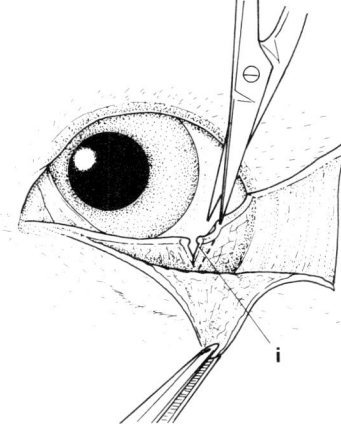

Fig. 6.18. Removal of the tarso-conjunctival wedge. (i) Wedge to be removed.

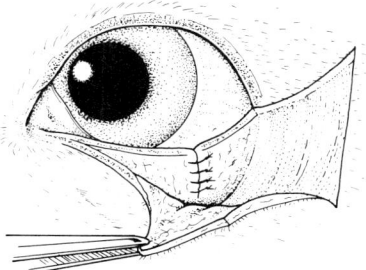

Fig. 6.19. The tarso-conjunctival tissue has been sutured.

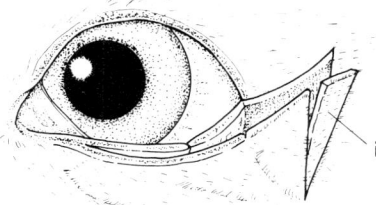

Fig. 6.20. Skin flap tension is adjusted by trimming (i).

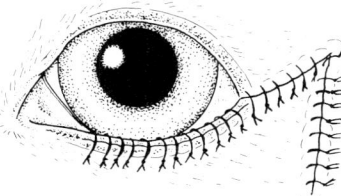

Fig. 6.21. Placement of the lid margin and skin sutures.

Partial tarsal plate excision for the correction of distichiasis

Indications

In distichiasis, extra cilia emerge from the eyelids via the Meibomian gland orifices or the margo–intermarginalis tissue (and occasionally the palpebral conjunctiva) to impinge upon the corneal surface. Trigeminal irritation is indicated by blepharospasm and epiphora, and both keratitis and corneal erosion can occur in severely affected patients.

Equipment

Scalpel with No. 15 disposable scalpel blade. Fine rat-tooth forceps. Distichiasis clamp.

Technique

Hair is clipped from the eyelid(s) and the skin prepared with Betadine solution.

The eyelid is held using the distichiasis clamp (Figs 6.22 and 6.24), and a 5 mm deep strip of cilia bearing distal tarsal plate tissue is removed using two parallel incisions along the margo–intermarginalis, the length of the defect (Figs 6.23 and 6.25). The wound is checked to make certain that all the root material has been removed, and scraped using the blunt edge of the scalpel should hair or root material still be visible in the tarsal plate tissue (Fig. 6.26). The wound is not sutured, but left to granulate so as to prevent any cicatricial distortion of the posterior eyelid margin. Cilia emerging from the palpebral conjunctiva are simply dissected out using a No. 11 scalpel blade.

Postoperative care

Topical antibiosis is used for 7 days.

Possible complications

Inaccurate dissection will lead to lid distortion and trichiasis.

Insufficient dissection will allow the re-emergence of the cilia.

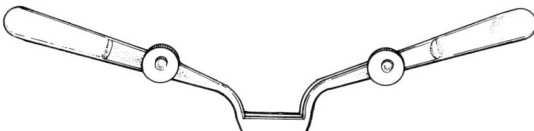

Fig. 6.22. Distichiasis clamp.

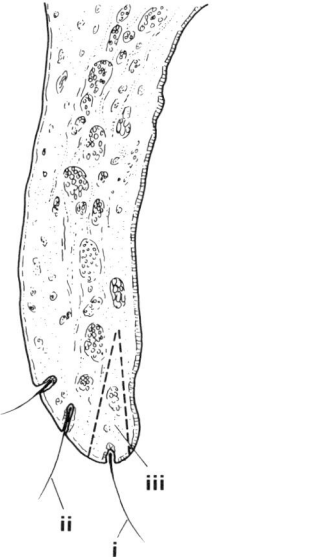

Fig. 6.23. Distichiasis. (a) The distichia; (b) normal lashes; (c) the wedge of tarsal plate tissue removed.

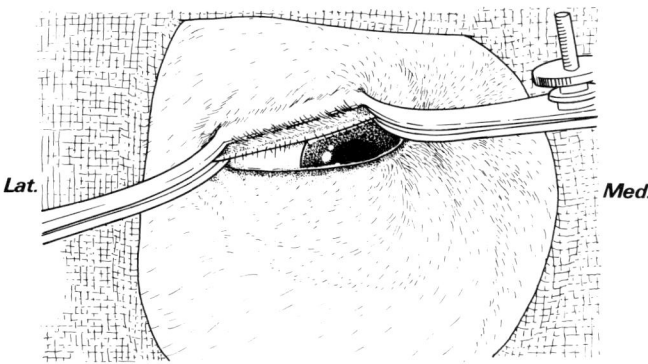

Fig. 6.24. The clamp has been applied to the upper right eyelid.

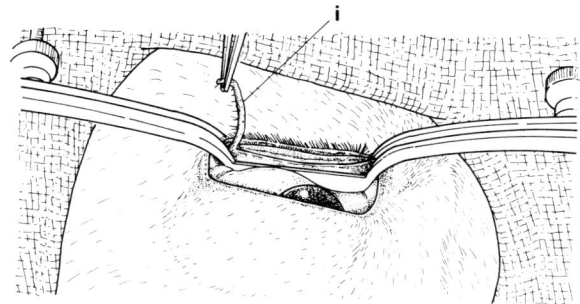

Fig. 6.25. The strip of tarsal plate tissue (i) is being removed.

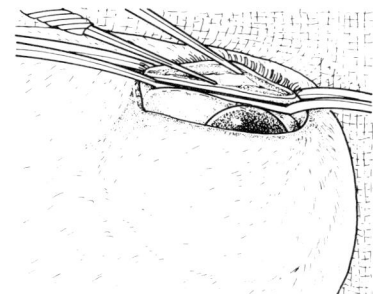

Fig. 6.26. The completed resection, the wound being examined for residual root material.

Full thickness vertical eyelid flap

Indication

The repair of the eyelid where the removal of neoplasia by the simple wedge resection techniques could result in post-operative distortion, with consequent corneal disease.

Equipment

Scalpel with a No. 15 blade, fine dissection scissors and fine rat-tooth forceps. The suture material used for the repair of the palpebral conjunctiva must be absorbable (polyglycolic acid, Dexon). Skin repair may be effected using absorbable or silk sutures, but the use of the former obviates suture removal from a difficult site in the conscious patient.

Technique

The removal of both benign and malignant eyelid neoplasia sometimes necessitates a full thickness resection of the eyelid (Fig. 6.27). The defect thus produced should be symmetrical, and all haemorrhage must be stopped before the repair is attempted. A palpebral conjunctival flap is mobilized from the loose conjunctival tissue distal to the surgical defect, and is sutured in position along its lateral edges using minimal 6-0 or 7-0 suture material (Fig. 6.28). The knots are tied in the conjunctival tissue to avoid corneal contact. A skin and muscle flap is then mobilized to fill the defect by extending the original lateral 'excision' incisions and removing two triangular wedges at the distal ends of these incisions (Fig. 6.29). This flap must be sufficiently large to fill the defect without tension. The flap is then advanced to fill the defect, covering the conjunctival flap, and the conjunctiva is then sutured to the skin along the 'new' eyelid margin (Fig. 6.30). The knots are tied to avoid corneal contact, and the skin incisions are closed in the usual way.

Postoperative care

Seven days systemic antibiosis is routine, and an occulentum is used to prevent corneal trauma by the conjunctival and marginal sutures. Self-trauma is prevented by the use of an Elizabethan collar.

Possible complications

Inadequate haemostasis can result in wound breakdown, and the use of too small a skin and muscle flap will result in the production of a cicatricial ectropion.

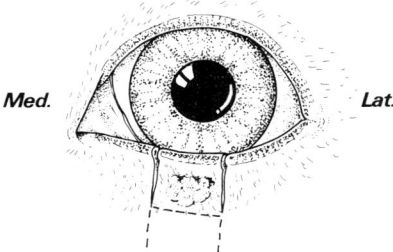

Fig. 6.27. Removal of the neoplastic tissue by full thickness resection.

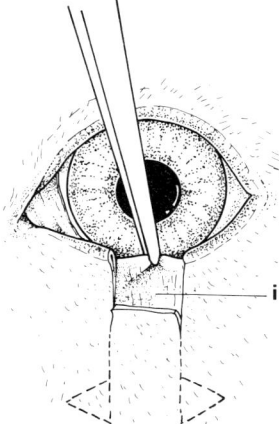

Fig. 6.28. Mobilization of the palpebral conjunctival flap. (i) The flap.

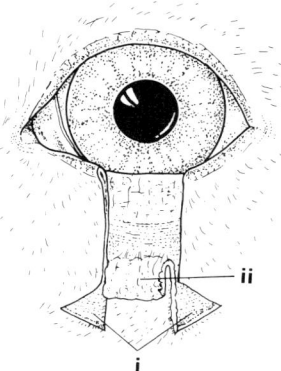

Fig. 6.29. Mobilization of the skin and muscle flap. (i) Triangular skin wedge resections; (ii) skin and muscle flap.

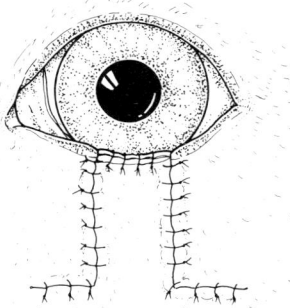

Fig. 6.30. The completed repair.

Conjunctival flaps

Indications

Indolent corneal ulcers, including those that have not responded to medical treatment; keratocoele; collagenase ulcer; to reduce pain and irritation associated with corneal wounds and ulcers; penetrating corneal wounds and lacerations; to cover the cornea in cases of severe eyelid damage; to cover the cornea in cases of facial nerve paralysis; eyeball proptosis; to protect the globe in cases of retrobulbar swelling following prolapse.

Conjunctival flaps promote healing and protect the cornea in all the above situations.

Equipment

Eyelid speculum, fine 2-in-1 rat-tooth forceps, small bluntly pointed scissors, small needle ($^3/_8$ inch), suitable suture material (fine braided nylon or silk, NOT monofilament nylon), needle holders.

Techniques

The membrana nictitans, or third eyelid, may be used as a type of ready-made conjunctival flap, therefore eliminating the surgery, albeit minor, associated with the preparation of either the fornix-based or limbal-based conjunctival flaps described below. General anaesthesia is preferable for all conjunctival flap techniques, but is not as essential (particularly in horses and cattle) for the membrana flap as the other two.

The eye should be carefully cleaned of any haemorrhage or discharge and in cases of indolent ulcers any dead corneal epithelium removed by chemical cauterization or other method. Any penetrating corneal wounds should first be sutured. In cases of prominent keratocoele a paracentesis may usefully be performed, through healthy cornea just inside the limbus and away from the lesion, via a shelving and short corneal incision which will not require suturing.

1 Membrana nictitans flap. About four single interrupted, or mattress, sutures are placed through the fleshy ridge, found just below or parallel to the free border of the outer aspect of the third eyelid (Figs 6.31 and 6.32), and to a fold of bulbar conjunctiva, behind the limbus, grasped with fine rat-tooth forceps (Figs. 6.33 and 6.34). These sutures should be loosely placed but the knots tightly tied, so reducing the possibility of them being pulled out or untied due to the constant eyelid and globe movements which occur in the conscious animal. These sutures pull the third eyelid over the globe and completely cover the cornea. The sutures should not go through the free border of the membrana as they will tend to pull out and leave a permanently ragged edge to the third eyelid.

An alternative method is to place the sutures through the upper lid (instead of the bulbar conjunctiva) and tie them to small buttons or pegs on the outside of the lid. In this latter method the membrana flap can be kept for a longer period, if desired, but there is always friction between the corneal surface and the inner aspect of the third eyelid with eyeball movement. This friction is eliminated in the first method described as the third eyelid, sutured to the bulbar conjunctiva, moves with eyeball movement.

The sutures are removed in about 1 week's time. It is usual for there to be some degree of corneal oedema present, but this will clear spontaneously within a few days. Rarely do adhesions occur between the cornea and the inner aspect of the third eyelid, unless this is deliberately scarified prior to suturing the flap.

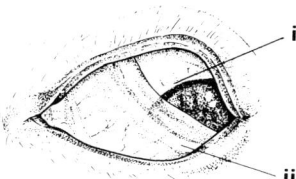

Fig. 6.31. Membrana nictitans exposed to show the fleshy ridge for suture placement. (i) Limbus; (ii) fleshy ridge.

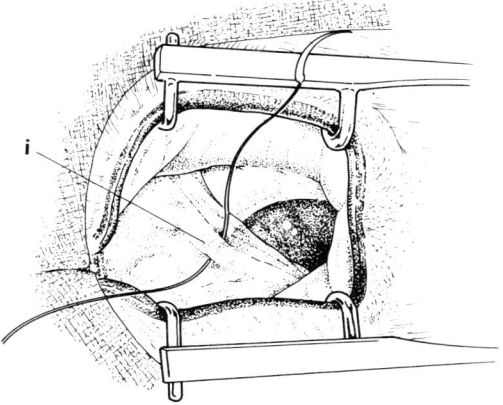

Fig. 6.32. Suture being placed through the fleshy ridge of membrana tissue (i).

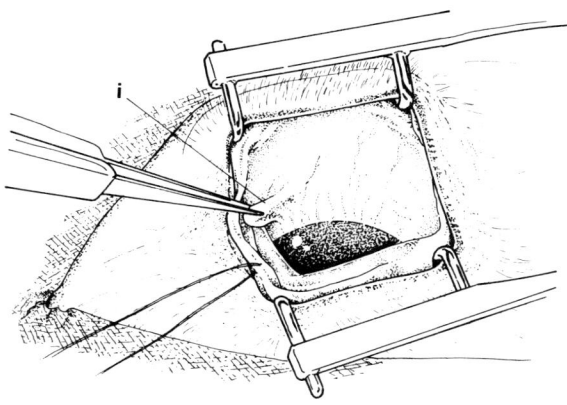

Fig. 6.33. Sutures are placed through the fold of bulbar conjunctiva (i).

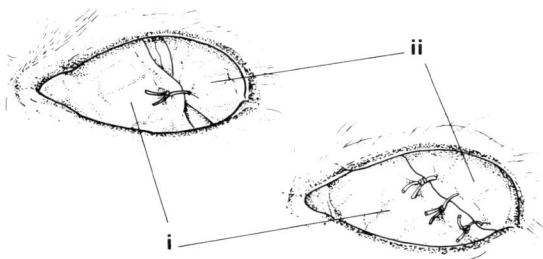

Fig. 6.34. Completing the suturing. (i) Membrana nictitans; (ii) bulbar conjunctiva.

2 Fornix-based flap. An incision is made through the bulbar conjunctiva, parallel to and immediately behind the limbus, for approximately one third of the circumference, using bluntly pointed scissors (Fig. 6.35). The flap is undermined by blunt dissection and then drawn over the cornea so that the raw or rough surface is in contact with the cornea (Fig. 6.36). The flap is anchored to the sclera (or bulbar conjunctiva) about 1 mm behind the opposite limbus, using three or four simple sutures. A lateral canthotomy will be helpful for additional exposure if this is required.

The fornix-based flap may be partial (covering only part of the cornea) or complete (covering the whole cornea). In the latter case some difficulty may be encountered in the area behind the nictitating membrane and separate superior and inferior flaps may be prepared and sutured together by mattress sutures.

The sutures can be removed 1 week to 10 days postoperatively. Adherence of the fornix-based flap to the corneal lesion is usual. In these cases the flap should be trimmed around the area of adherence when atrophy of the remaining conjunctiva will occur.

3 Limbal-based flap. In this type of flap, the incision is made in the conjunctiva some distance from the limbus, i.e. towards the limit of the bulbar conjunctiva near the fornix (Fig. 6.37), and at each end of the flap the incision is extended down to the limbus. Small bluntly pointed scissors are again used and the flap undermined by blunt dissection down to the limbus, taking care not to incise through the flap base. The flap is then turned over the cornea so that the outer, smooth, conjunctival surface is in apposition to the cornea (Fig. 6.38), i.e. the opposite to the fornix-based flap. The flap is then anchored to the lower limbus as before.

Removal of the sutures is 1 week to 10 days later; adhesion to the cornea is rare.

Postoperative care

Provided that some soft suture material is used and the sutures loosely laid but the knots tightly tied, self-inflicted damage does not occur and Elizabethan collars are unnecessary. Care should be taken that the flap does not exert pressure on the cornea, and this may occur if the width of the flap is too narrow.

Medical therapy, e.g. atropine and/or antibiotic may be continued postoperatively if desired.

Possible complications

The only possible complication encountered using any of these flaps is if the sutures pull out, in which case they may be replaced. This should not occur if the precautions mentioned above are taken.

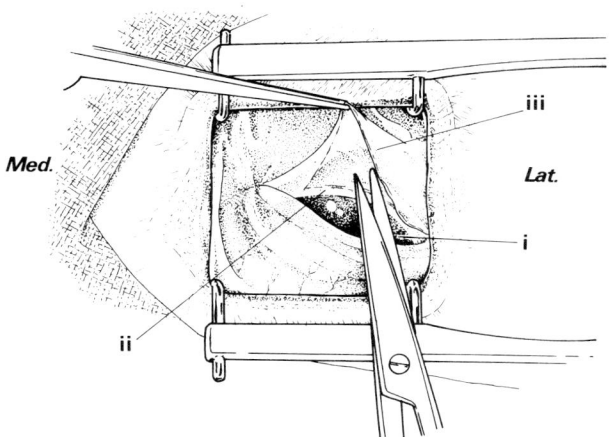

Fig. 6.35. Dissection of the bulbar conjunctiva. (i) Limbus; (ii) line of incision; (iii) dissected conjunctiva.

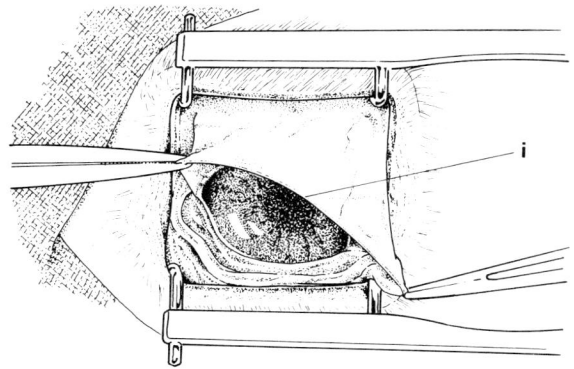

Fig. 6.36. The conjunctival flap (i) is being drawn down over the corneal surface.

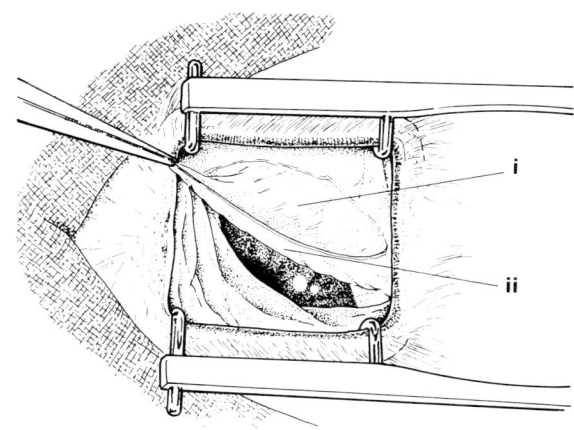

Fig. 6.37. The bulbar conjunctiva is incised parallel to and well behind the limbus. (i) Subconjunctival/Tenon's capsule tissue; (ii) the conjunctival flap.

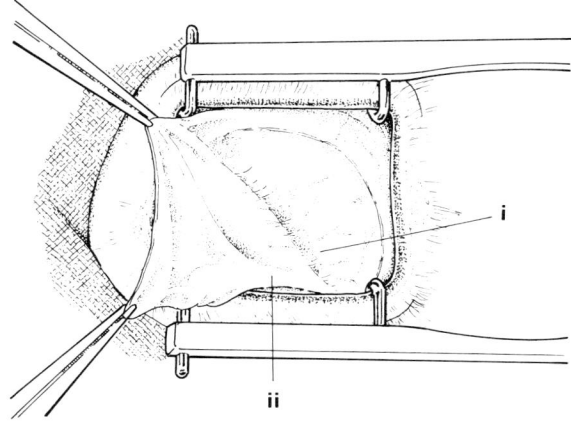

Fig. 6.38. The conjunctiva has been undermined forwards to the limbus. (i) Line of the limbus seen through the conjunctival tissue; (ii) the conjunctival flap.

Parotid duct transposition

Indication

Keratoconjunctivitis sicca or 'dry eye'.

Equipment

One piece of black monofilament nylon (Size 5) and a fine pair of rat-tooth forceps for duct cannulation. Small scalpel and selection of fine scissors and small plain and rat-tooth forceps, mosquito forceps, 6-0 plain collagen and skin suture materials, needle holders.

Technique

General anaesthesia

The opening of the parotid duct is to be found in the mouth on the end of a prominent papilla, opposite the carnassial tooth, just beyond the reflection of mucous membrane onto the cheek. The piece of monofilament nylon is carefully inserted through the opening and, sometimes with a little difficulty, is introduced into the duct and gently pushed as far back as possible (Fig. 6.39). The end of the nylon is cut off leaving about ½ inch showing. (Do not confuse the parotid opening with the opening of the zygomatic salivary gland which is slightly posterior and nearer to the gum margin.)

After the usual shaving, skin preparation and draping of the site, a horizontal incision is made through the skin in the area between the lower lid and upper lip and about one third distance below the lid, extending from the medial canthus backwards to a distance of about one-and-a-half times the width of the palpebral fissure (Fig. 6.40).

Via the skin incision, the nylon-cannulated parotid duct is located by blunt dissection through paniculus muscle taking care not to damage the overlying facial nerve and vein. The presence of the nylon within the duct renders identification easy. The duct is lifted and roughly dissected free from other tissue, working anteriorly towards its opening into the mouth (Fig. 6.41). It is wise not to remove too much connective tissue from around the parotid duct. When the duct has been traced as far forwards as its opening into the mouth, an incision is made through the buccal mucosa, from inside the cheek, and into the mouth, freeing the papilla from the rest of the oral mucous membrane (Fig. 6.42). Great care should be taken not to cut into the papilla and it is good policy to remove a surrounding piece of mucous membrane as this can easily be trimmed prior to insertion of the papilla into the lower conjunctival sac. The opening into the mouth is then closed with simple, interrupted absorbable sutures placed from inside the cheek. The parotid duct and papilla can be further freed towards the parotid gland if necessary, which will be the case if there is any tension on the duct when the papilla is placed in the conjunctival sac.

The parotid papilla is sutured into the lower conjunctival sac, located by blunt dissection just below the rim of the lower part of the bony orbit (Fig. 6.43). It is better placed in the lateral part so that it is not involved with the nictitating membrane attachments. It is quite unnecessary to place it in the upper conjunctival fornix; this complicates the operation and necessitates freeing more of the parotid duct posteriorly. The conjunctival sac is recognized by putting a pair of artery forceps into it via the palpebral orifice. A small piece of the conjunctival sac is then tented up by holding with two pairs of mosquito forceps from inside the facial wound. This piece of conjunctival sac is then incised and the opening checked to ensure that it enters the conjunctival sac by pushing a pair of forceps through. The papilla is then sutured into place using 6-0 absorbable sutures placed at 12, 3, 6 and 9 o'clock, in such a way that the duct opening on the papilla is directly into the conjunctival sac and the knots are outside the sac and inside the facial wound (Fig. 6.44). Before placing the last of these four sutures the piece of monofilament nylon is withdrawn. Further sutures are put around the junction between the papilla and the conjunctival sac to prevent escape of parotid fluid into the wound.

The transposition is now complete and the skin facial wound closed in the conventional manner.

Postoperative care

Transposition of the parotid duct papilla from the mouth, through the cheek and into the conjunctival sac, however efficient the surgical technique, must carry some danger of infection and a course of postoperative broad-spectrum antibiotic is indicated. (In spite of this obvious danger, no case of postoperative infection has ever been encountered following this operation.)

The eye is carefully cleaned the morning following surgery, although this procedure is likely to be far less necessary than was the case prior to operation. It is probably advisable during the first few postoperative days to divide the food intake into several small meals, as this will ensure the flow of parotid secretion.

Possible complications

As has been stated, infection of the wound has never been a problem, but some swelling of the face is likely for a few days following surgery, particularly in those breeds in which there is little subcutaneous tissue on the side of the face.

A wet eye in place of a dry eye is a very definite postoperative complication, and the deposition of a fine grey film on the cornea due to the parotid secretion occurs in some cases. However, this operation undoubtedly relieves the necessity for the frequent cleaning of the unpleasant, purulent-like, tacky, and often profuse, discharge and the constant use of a false tear preparation which accompanies all cases of keratoconjunctivitis sicca.

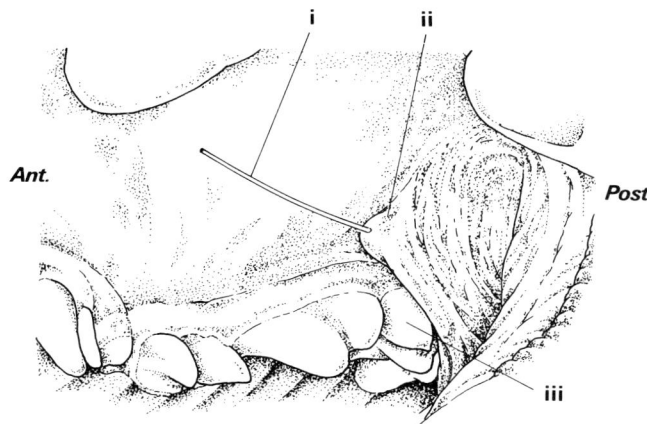

Fig. 6.39. Cannulation of the parotid duct with nylon, showing the position of the papilla in relation to the carnassial tooth. (i) Monofilament nylon; (ii) parotid papilla; (iii) carnassial tooth.

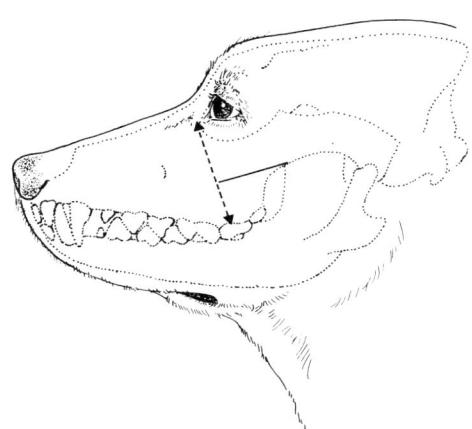

Fig. 6.40. The length and position of the skin incision.

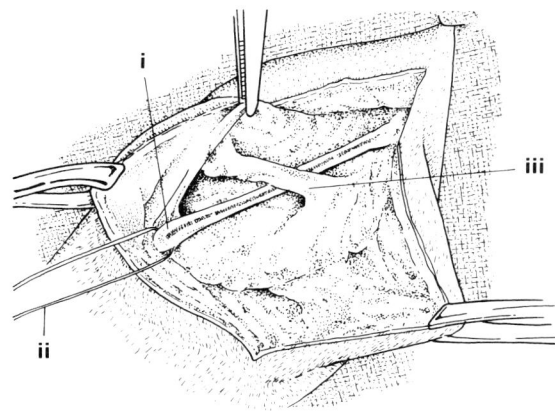

Fig. 6.41. The partially dissected parotid duct, lying beneath the facial nerve. (i) The cannulated duct; (ii) suture material being used to elevate the duct to facilitate the dissection; (iii) the facial nerve.

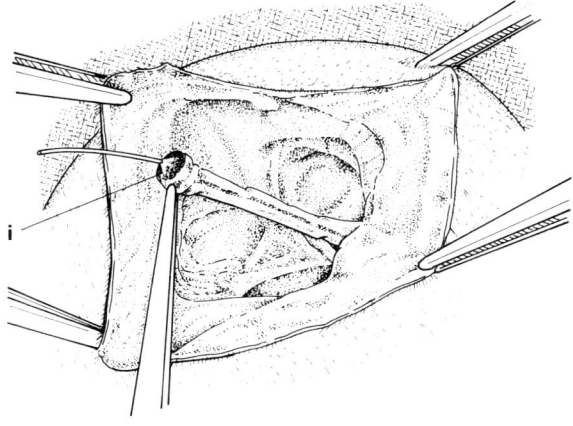

Fig. 6.42. The papilla (i) has been dissected free from the buccal mucosa.

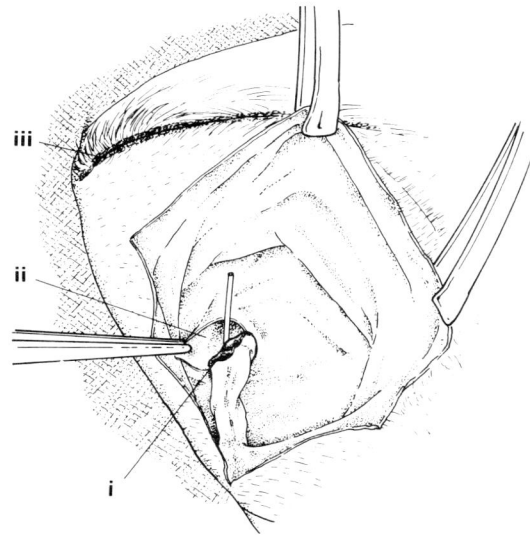

Fig. 6.43. The papilla (i) and duct are being passed under the facial skin to the lower conjunctival sac. (ii) Is the tunnel to the conjunctival sac and (iii) the palpebral fissure.

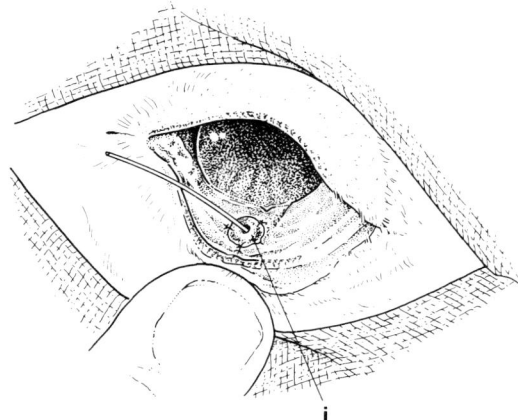

Fig. 6.44. The papilla has been sutured into the lower conjunctival sac.

Superficial keratectomy

Indications

The removal of any anterior corneal stromal opacitation to improve vision. The technique may thus be used in the treatment of corneal cholesterolosis, corneal degeneration, pannus (chronic superficial keratitis), traumatic corneal scarring, and keratitis pigmentosa.

Equipment

Scalpel with a No. 15 blade, fine dissection scissors and fine rat-tooth forceps.

Technique

The circumorbital hair is removed by clipping and the skin prepared using Betadine solution.

A lateral canthotomy may be necessary to expose the cornea adequately. The area of corneal opacitation, which may involve the whole of the corneal surface area, is removed by cutting into the thickness of the cornea to a level deeper than the opacity, and then splitting the corneal stroma between its lamellae to remove the diseased tissue (Fig. 6.45). The technique may be likened to the removal of the outer layer of an onion.

Small opacities are removed in one piece, the incision starting over the corneal surface and dissecting outwards to the limbus. The corneal segment may then be detached using the scalpel or the dissecting scissors. Large opacities are best removed in two or three pieces, whilst a total superficial keratectomy is best effected using a limbus-to-limbus cruciate incision and peeling back the four segments from the central cornea (Figs. 6.46 and 6.47). A membrana nictitans flap should be used to cover the larger keratectomy wounds for 2 weeks to facilitate epithelialization and reduce the chance of infection.

Postoperative care

Topical antibiosis for 2–3 weeks, or until epithelialization has been completed, is essential. Topical and possible subconjunctival corticosteroid therapy must be used to reduce the amount of corneal vascularization and the tendency towards the production of granulation and scar tissue, particularly with the larger wounds. The patient usually experiences no apparent discomfort following keratectomy with or without membrana flapping, but an Elizabethan collar will prevent any self-trauma.

Possible complications

Deep dissection of the cornea may lead to anterior chamber penetration at the time of surgery, or globe rupture during the postoperative phase. Healing by epithelialization with a minimum of, or no, vascularization is achieved by sufficiency of the corticosteroid therapy, an insufficiency leading to a loss of corneal transparency by scar tissue formation.

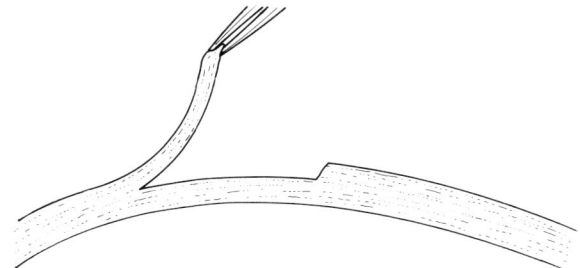

Fig. 6.45. Schematic representation of superficial keratectomy.

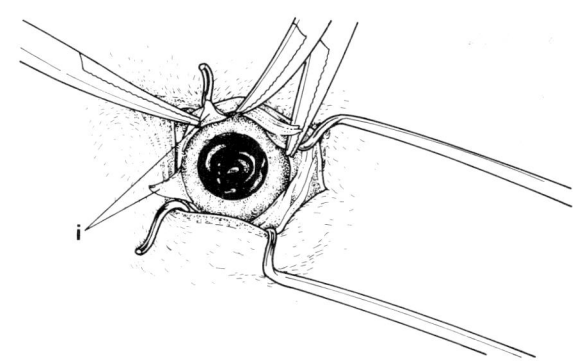

Fig. 6.47. Total superficial keratectomy: the completed dissection, with the two medial quadrants only attached at the limbus (i).

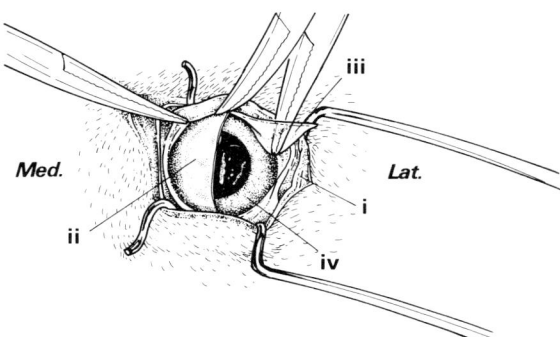

Fig. 6.46. Total superficial keratectomy: 50% of the diseased tissue has been removed. (i) Lateral canthotomy; (ii) opaque cornea; (iii) a quadrant of opaque cornea being removed; (iv) iris.

Enucleation

Indications

Removal of the globe is indicated primarily for the humane relief of intractable pain and discomfort. Chronic glaucoma and hydrophthalmos. Chronic ocular inflammation and infection. Extensive laceration and perforating injury to the eye. Prolonged exposure following prolapse. Serious optic nerve and extra-ocular muscle injury following prolapse. Phthisis bulbi with secondary entropion, conjunctivitis and keratitis. In circumstances where the temperament of the animal or the circumstances of the owner render necessary medical therapy impossible.

Equipment

A general surgical pack, incorporating Allis tissue forceps, fine curved scissors, a long curved haemostat and small 1/2 and 3/8 curved cutting needles.

Technique

The lid edges are closed in a natural fashion and two pairs of Allis forceps used to clamp the margins in apposition closing the conjunctival sac.

An incision is made through the skin of both upper and lower lids 3–4 mm from the lid margins. These incisions meet beyond the medial and lateral canthus (Fig. 6.48). Care is taken not to damage the branches of the angular vein adjacent to the medial canthus.

The line of incision is deepened using sharp and blunt dissection, subcutaneous fascia and orbicularis muscle is cut. The extent of the conjunctival sac is recognized and its puncture is studiously avoided (Fig. 6.49).

Blunt dissection and finger-tip palpation reveals the bony margin of the orbit. The periorbital fascia is tensioned by traction on the Allis forceps and is sectioned within the orbital margin releasing the globe and allowing it to be drawn outwards. Lateral traction of the globe allows identification of both the medial and lateral canthus 'ligaments' which are carefully sectioned as they become taut (Fig. 6.49).

The globe is drawn further from the orbit and as it is rotated the insertions of the extraocular muscles upon it are recognized and cut as close to the globe as possible with fine curved scissors (Fig. 6.50). The position of the optic nerve is now identified as a tense cord. If conformation allows, a ligature of size 0 gut may be placed around the nerve and associated blood vessels before it is sectioned with scissors close to the posterior pole. Otherwise, the jaws of a curved haemostat are passed around the globe and clamped onto the nerve so as to leave a stump of sufficient length for the placement of a ligature following section of the nerve. If there is insufficient space a transfixion ligature may be employed by passing the suture through the retractor muscle before tying it. Inevitably there are cases in which haemostasis must rely on crushing the stump with forceps. The globe can now be withdrawn, together with the attached lid edges, conjunctival sac, third eyelid and associated fascia.

Some bleeding within the orbit is to be expected. It is controlled by packing as firmly as possible with gauze swabs but has often not ceased when closure of the orbit is commenced.

Primary closure consists of drawing together within the orbit a pad of extraocular muscle and fascia with single interrupted sutures of 3-0 gut carried on a small ½ or ³/₈ curved cutting needle to facilitate manipulation within the orbit. Suture ends are cut short. A second layer of closure is completed by grasping the soft tissues and fascia at the dorsal and ventral margin of the orbit and drawing it towards the horizontal midline where it is retained by a series of interrupted gut sutures (Fig. 6.51).

Closure of the skin wound is preceded by careful trimming of strips of skin from the wound edge with straight scissors so that the incision may be neatly closed with 4-0 monofilament nylon or 3-0 Supramid without any redundant folding.

Postoperative care

Systemic broad spectrum antibiotics are used for 5 days postoperatively.

Possible complications

The major surgical complication is excessive haemorrhage into the orbit obscuring the surgical field. This problem may be anticipated and largely overcome by care in dissection within the orbit and avoiding trauma to intraorbital soft tissue, avoiding stripping the retractor muscle sheath from the optic nerve, sectioning tendons rather than extraocular muscular tissue and giving special attention to the early ligation or crushing of the optic nerve and its sheath of muscle.

Forceful packing of the orbit with swabs for a short time around the haemostat placed upon the nerve and muscle stump will normally provide a site in which closure can be resumed.

Discharge via the suture line is rare. It is treated by creating a drainage pathway by blunt probing of the orbit and evacuating the contents by massage and irrigation with antibiotics indicated by culture. This may be followed by curettage or the removal of infected tissue and suture materials following reopening of the original wound.

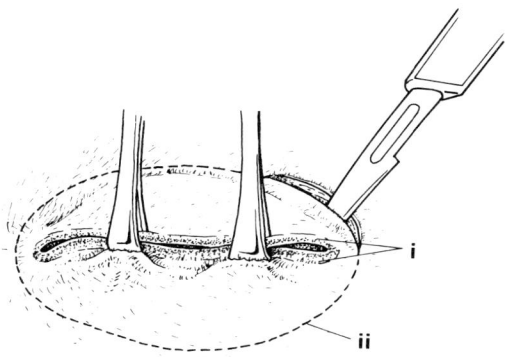

Fig. 6.48. Clamping the lid margins and the skin incisions. (i) The closed lid edges; (ii) the line of incision.

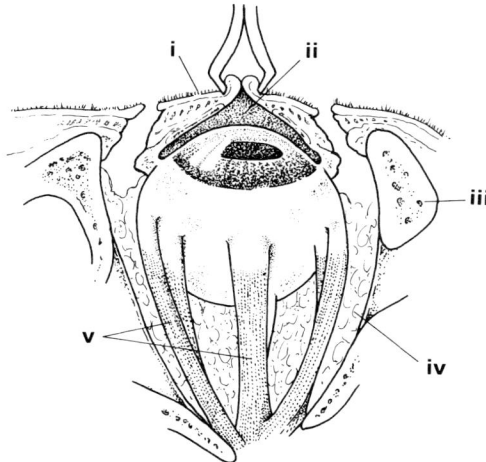

Fig. 6.49. Incision of the skin and fascia. (i) Lower eyelid; (ii) conjunctival sac; (iii) orbital ridge; (iv) adipose tissue; (v) extra ocular muscles.

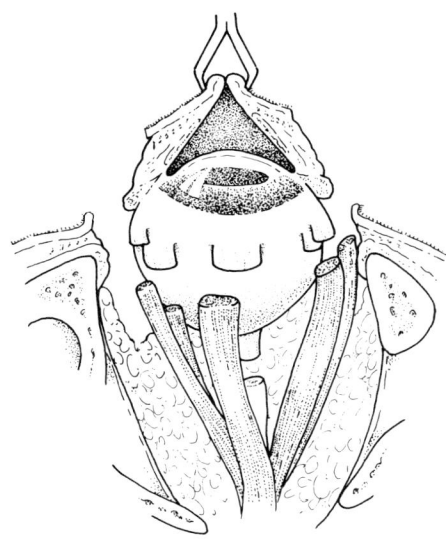

Fig. 6.50. Section of the extraocular muscles and optic nerve.

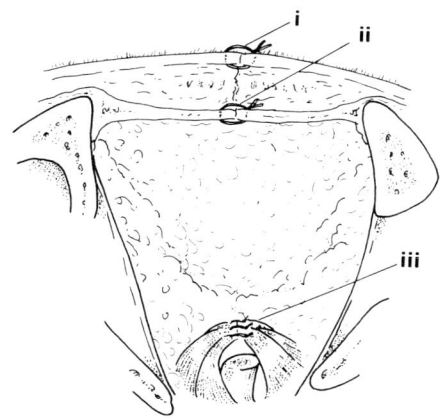

Fig. 6.51. The layers of repair. (a) Sutured skin; (b) sutured fascia; (c) sutured stumps of extraocular muscles.

Chapter 7
Orthopaedic Surgery

HAMISH R. DENNY

Shoulder arthrotomy

Indication

Treatment of osteochondritis dissecans.

Equipment

A routine surgical set plus a Hohmann retractor, a Traver's retractor, a St Thomas pattern elevator and a Sim's uterine curette.

Technique

A skin incision is made over the distal third of the scapular spine and extended over the shoulder and proximal third of the humeral shaft. Subcutaneous fat and fascia are retracted (Fig. 7.1). The acromion and the proximal end of the acromial head of the deltoid muscle lie beneath a thin sheet of muscle, the omotransversarius; this muscle is reflected (Fig. 7.2). The blades of a curved pair of scissors are introduced under the origin of the deltoid (Fig. 7.3) and the muscle is transected with a scalpel approximately 2 cm from the acromion. The muscle is reflected to reveal the infraspinatus and teres minor muscles (Fig. 7.4). The two muscle bellies are separated with a self-retaining retractor (Traver's or West's) to reveal the joint capsule. A horizontal incision is made in the capsule. The joint surfaces are separated with the aid of a Hohmann retractor to expose the osteochondritis dissecans lesion which normally lies in the caudal surface of the humeral head (Fig. 7.5). The lesion generally consists of a cartilaginous flap, 1–2 cm in diameter, which covers an erosion in the subchondral bone. The free edge of the flap is grasped with artery forceps, a periosteal elevator (St Thomas pattern) is slipped beneath the flap and used to break the medial attachments. Once the cartilaginous flap has been removed the edges of the subchondral erosion are curetted (Sim's uterine curette) unless the erosion appears to be healing and is filling with fibrocartilage. Occasionally the cartilaginous flap will break off as the joint is levered open and fall into the caudal or medial compartment, which can make retrieval difficult. However, flexion, extension and rotation of the joint a few times will generally cause the fragment to float up into the arthrotomy incision for removal.

The joint capsule, if easily accessible, is repaired with simple interrupted sutures of linen or fine monofilament nylon. However, if difficulty is experienced it is sufficient to coapt the muscle bellies of the infraspinatus and teres minor with a continuous catgut suture to seal the joint capsule. The transected acromial head of the deltoid is repaired with mattress sutures of linen thread or monofilament nylon. The subcutaneous fascia is coapted with a continuous catgut suture and the skin with mattress sutures of monofilament nylon.

The surgical approach described above gives good exposure and is recommended for the surgeon who only occasionally performs shoulder surgery. A less traumatic approach is recommended for more experienced surgeons. Instead of transecting the acromial head of the deltoid the infraspinatus and teres minor muscles are exposed by separation of the acromial and scapular heads of the deltoid muscle.

Postoperative care

Antibiotic cover is provided for 5 days, skin sutures are removed at 10 days and exercise is restricted for 4 weeks. Full limb function is usually regained within 3 months of surgery. In dogs with bilateral lesions, a 6 week interval is left between each arthrotomy and the second operation is only performed if the dog is lame on the contralateral leg.

Possible complications

1 Excessive muscle damage during exposure and possibly failure to close the joint capsule may lead to seroma formation within a few days of surgery. Needle aspiration of the seroma is carried out as necessary.
2 Skin overlying the shoulder joint is very mobile, wound healing may be slower than normal and skin sutures are left *in situ* for at least 10 days to avoid the risk of wound breakdown.

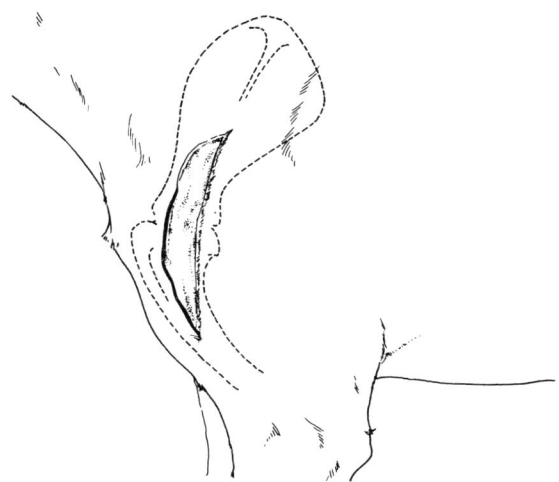

Fig. 7.1. The site of incision.

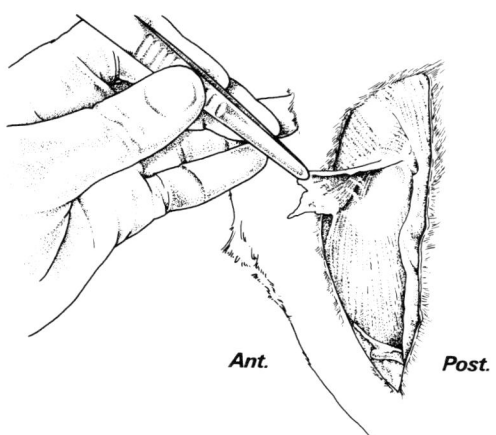

Ant. **Post.**

Fig. 7.2. Reflection of the omotransversarius muscle.

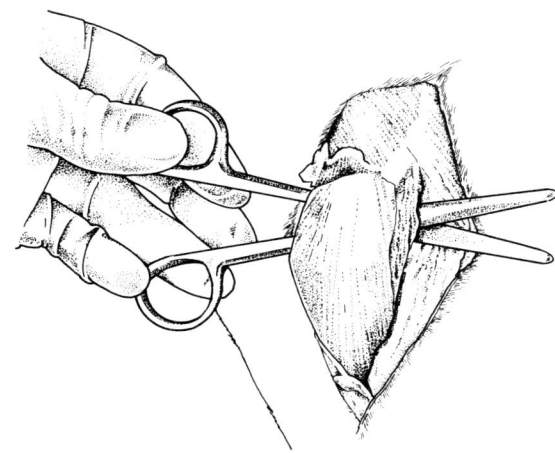

Fig. 7.3. The origin of the deltoid muscle.

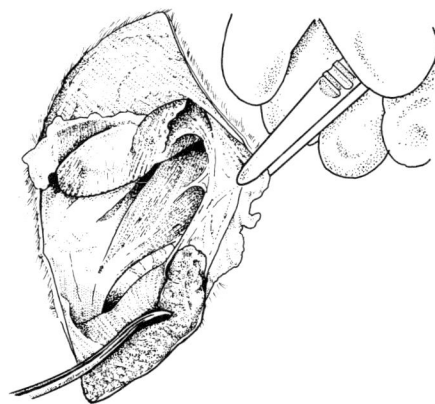

Fig. 7.4. Transection of the deltoid to reveal the infraspinatus and teres minor muscle.

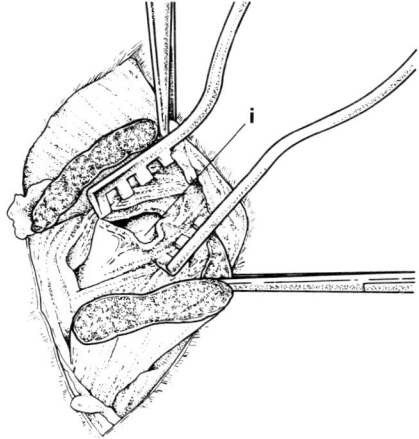

Fig. 7.5. The capsular incision (i).

Elbow — caudolateral arthrotomy

Indication

Excision of an ununited anconeal process.

Equipment

A routine surgical set plus a West's retractor and a St Thomas pattern elevator.

Technique

A skin incision is made along the caudal border of the lateral condyle of the humerus (Fig. 7.6). The fascia is incised along the cranial edge of the lateral head of the triceps and the muscle is retracted to expose the anconeus muscle. The anconeus muscle, together with the joint capsule to which it is closely attached, are incised just caudal to the lateral condyle (Fig. 7.7) (leaving sufficient muscle on the condylar side to be sutured later). A West's Retractor is used to separate the muscle edges and allow exposure of the caudal joint surfaces (Fig. 7.8). The elbow is flexed to reveal the anconeal process which is prised away from its cartilaginous attachments to the ulna with a periosteal elevator and removed.

The anconeus muscle and joint capsule are closed together with a continuous catgut suture and subsequent wound closure is routine.

Postoperative care

A support bandage is applied for a week postoperatively. Antibiotic cover is given for 5 days and skin sutures are removed at 10 days. Exercise is restricted for 4 weeks and then gradually increased. In dogs with bilateral lesions a 6-week interval is left between each arthrotomy. Normal limb function should be regained within 2 months of surgery.

Possible complications

The anconeal process normally contributes to the stability of the elbow joint. Instability after removal may predispose the dog to intermittent elbow sprains and osteoarthrosis. Grøndalen & Rørvik (1980) in a follow-up of thirty-seven dogs treated for ununited anconeal process reported 39% of cases were occasionally lame after hard exercise or were stiff after rest.

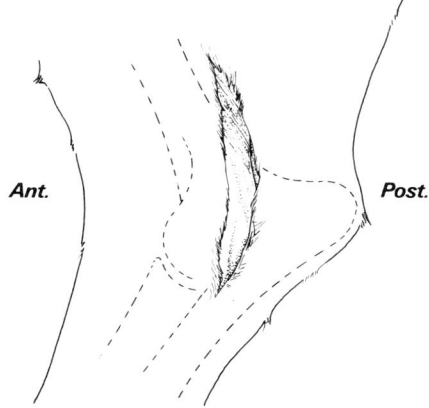

Fig. 7.6. The site of incision.

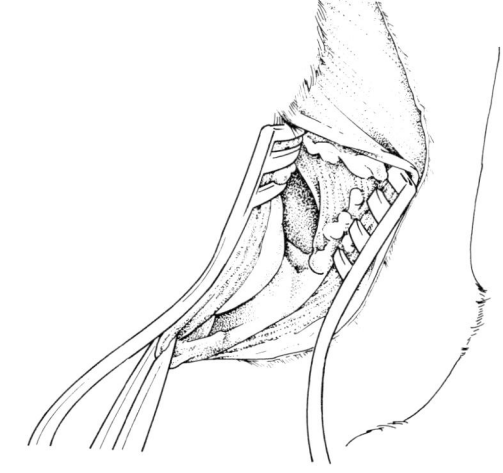

Fig. 7.8. Exposure of the joint surfaces.

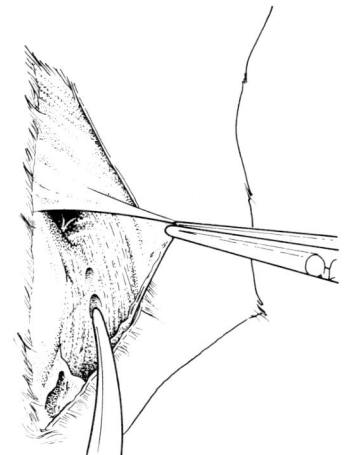

Fig. 7.7. Incision of anconeus muscle and joint capsule.

Elbow—medial arthrotomy

Indications

The surgical treatment of osteochondritis dissecans and the removal of ununited coronoid process.

Early diagnosis is important—these conditions result in osteoarthrosis and surgery should be carried out before joint changes become advanced.

Equipment

A routine surgical set plus a West's retractor, two Hohmann retractors, and a Volkmann's double-ended curette.

Technique

After routine surgical preparation the dog is placed on its side and a bolster is placed beneath the elbow. A skin incision is made over the medial humeral condyle (Fig. 7.9). The pronator teres and flexor carpi radialis muscles are separated close to their origin on the medial epicondyle and retracted with a West's retractor. A vertical incision is made into the joint capsule over the humeral condyle only (Fig. 7.10). The blades of a pair of straight scissors are then introduced between the articular surfaces of the joint and spread laterally to complete exposure (Fig. 7.11). The West's retractor is repositioned to include the cut edges of the joint capsule. This method of arthrotomy minimizes the risk of damage to the median nerve and artery which cross the anterior and distal margins of the joint. The articular surfaces are separated with the aid of Hohmann retractors and exposure is improved with the aid of an assistant who exerts pressure on the forearm and 'hinges' the elbow over the bolster (Fig. 7.12).

The medial condyle of the humerus is inspected for an osteochondritis dissecans lesion. If a cartilaginous flap is present, it is removed and the underlying erosion in the subchondral bone is curetted. In some cases the lesion takes the form of fissures in the cartilage this area is curetted. If there is no evidence of osteochondritis dissecans the coronoid process is inspected, free from any remaining cartilaginous or fibrous attachments and removed. The coronoid process will be found either as a discrete triangular fragment of bone and cartilage or it may be in the form of two or three fragments. The coronoid process lies immediately beneath the medial collateral ligament and exposure can be improved by cutting the caudal margin of the collateral ligament, however complete section of the ligament should not be necessary.

Osteochondritis dissecans and ununited coronoid process have the same aetiology (Olsson 1975) and consequently it is wise to inspect the coronoid process even when there is an obvious osteochondritis dissecans lesion present as both conditions can co-exist. After the lesion has been dealt with, the joint is flushed out with saline. The muscle bellies are coapted with a continuous suture of catgut which effectively seals the joint capsule. The rest of the wound closure is carried out in routine fashion.

Postoperative care

The elbow is supported with a bandage for 1 week. Antibiotic cover is given for 5 days and skin sutures are removed at 7 days. Exercise is restricted for 4 weeks and then gradually increased. In dogs with bilateral lesions, a 6-week interval is left between operations. Normal limb function is generally regained within 2 months of surgery and subsequent follow up reveals little increase in the degree of osteoarthritis present at the time of surgery (Denny & Gibbs 1980).

Possible complications

Osteoarthrosis present at the time of surgery or secondary to surgical interference may lead to poor exercise tolerance with varying degrees of lameness and a limited range of elbow movement.

Surgical exposure of the osteochondritis dissecans lesion or ununited coronoid process in the elbow can be difficult for the inexperienced surgeon and failure to identify and treat either lesion will result in progressive osteoarthrosis.

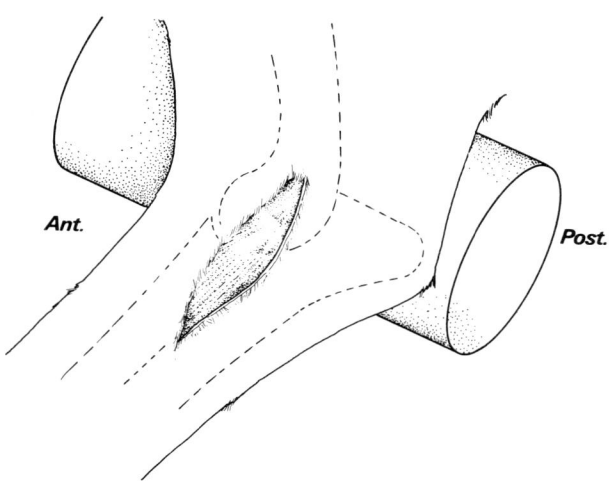

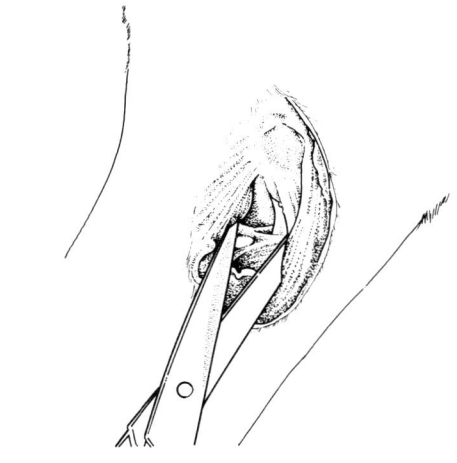

Fig. 7.11. Increasing the exposure.

Fig. 7.9. The site of incision.

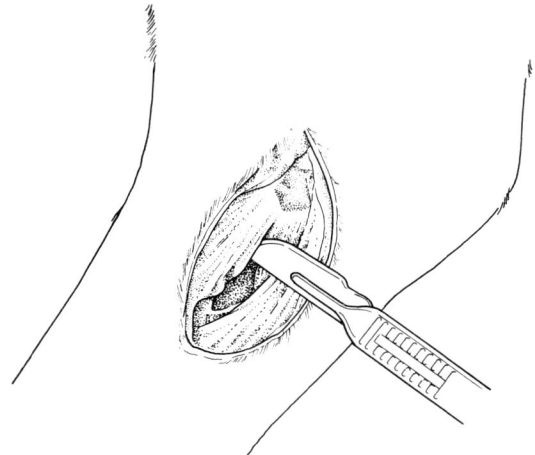

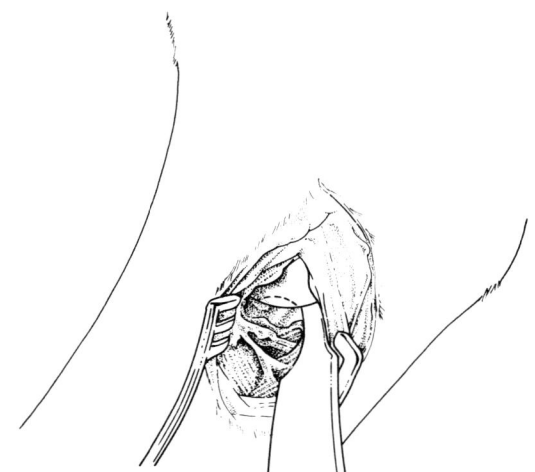

Fig. 7.10. Incision of the joint capsule.

Fig. 7.12. The completed exposure.

The hip toggle procedure

Indications

Recurrent or longstanding (up to 2 months) dislocations of the hip joint.

Equipment

A routine surgical set plus a Universal bone drill, drill bits ($^7/_{64}$ths and $^3/_{16}$ths diameter), Burn's bone holding forceps, two Hohmann retractors, a Traver's retractor, and a toggle constructed from a Kirschner wire (arthrodesis 0.045×5.0 inches, see Fig. 7.13). A double strand of No. 7 braided nylon is threaded through the loop of the toggle.

Technique

A skin incision is made directly over the greater trochanter and continued distally over the femur to the midshaft region (Fig. 7.14). The fascia lata is separated from the biceps femoris muscle using scissors. The biceps femoris is retracted to reveal the greater trochanter. The sciatic nerve is identified caudal to the femoral shaft in the loose fascia between the biceps femoris and the semimembranosus muscle. The path of the nerve is traced proximally around the hip (Fig. 7.15). The nerve is carefully protected while exposure of the acetabulum is completed from the caudal aspect. The insertion of the superficial gluteal muscle is transected and the caudal muscles of the hip (obturator and gemelli) if not already ruptured, are transected close to their insertion on the proximal femur (Figs 7.15 and 7.16). These muscles are reflected and the dislocated femoral head is retracted cranial to the acetabulum with bone-holding forceps applied to the proximal femoral shaft. Torn joint capsule is trimmed back and the acetabulum is cleared of haematoma or granulation tissue. When a pseudoarthrosis has formed in a long standing dislocation, thickened joint capsule must be removed and adhesions between the femoral head and dorsal rim of the acetabulum broken down before reduction of the dislocation can be achieved.

Once the acetabulum has been debrided, a tunnel is drilled through the acetabular fossa using a $^3/_{16}$ inch drill bit (Fig. 7.17). Artery forceps are used to guide the toggle into the tunnel then the blunt end of the $^7/_{64}$ inch drill bit is used to push the toggle completely through the acetabulum (Fig. 7.18a). Traction is applied to the braided nylon round ligament prosthesis to ensure that the toggle rotates and engages firmly on the medial side of the acetabulum (Fig. 7.18b).

The femoral head is rotated in a caudolateral direction. The blade of a Hohmann retractor is inserted between the caudal border of the gluteal muscles and the femoral neck. The retractor is used to elevate the femoral head out of the incision and remnants of the round ligament are removed. A second Hohmann retractor may be necessary to depress the biceps femoris muscle while a tunnel is drilled using $^7/_{64}$ inch bit from the fovea capitis through the femoral head and neck to emerge just ventral to the greater trochanter (Figs 7.19a and b). A second tunnel is drilled through the greater trochanter (Fig. 7.19b). Wire loops are placed through both tunnels. The braided nylon is drawn through the femoral tunnel using a loop. Traction is maintained on the nylon while the dislocation is reduced. Half the nylon is drawn through the trochanteric tunnel using the remaining wire loop and the free ends of the prosthesis are tightly tied. Reduction and stability of the hip should be checked before cutting off the excess nylon. Once reduction is complete, the obturator and gemellus muscles are no longer easily accessible and are left unsutured. The transected superficial gluteal muscle is repaired using horizontal mattress sutures of linen or fine monofilament nylon. The fascia lata and biceps femoris, the subcutaneous fascia and skin are coapted in layers in routine fashion.

Postoperative care

Antibiotic cover is provided for 5 days and skin sutures are generally removed after 8 days. Exercise is severely restricted for 4 weeks postoperatively.

Possible complications

1   Redislocation with rupture of the braided nylon round ligament prosthesis. Factors predisposing to premature breakage of the prosthesis include overactivity in the recovery period, hip dysplasia and muscle contraction in longstanding dislocations. The hip joint may be salvaged by excision of the femoral head.

2   If dislocation occurs in an immature dog before closure of the proximal femoral growth plate, then rupture of the joint capsule may lead to ischaemic necrosis of the femoral head. When this complication arises following the hip toggle procedure, excision arthroplasty should be carried out.

3   Osteoarthritis—this is a possible complication of any joint injury.

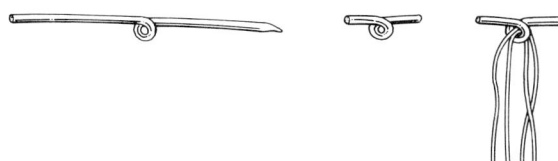

Fig. 7.13. The toggle.

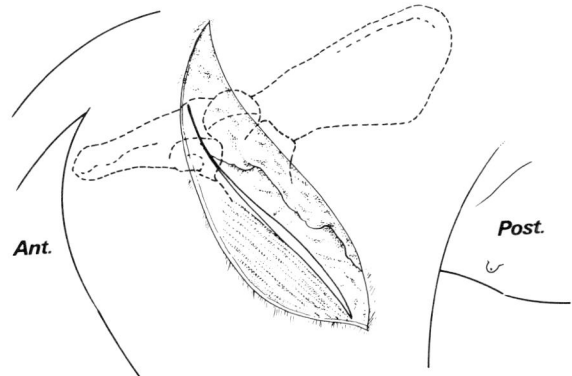

Fig. 7.14. The site of incision.

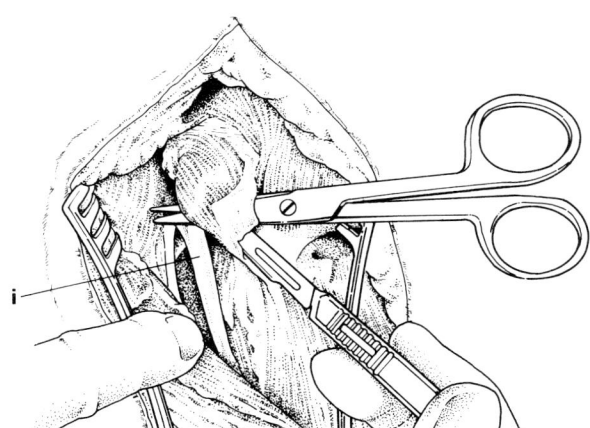

Fig. 7.15. Transection of the insertion of the superficial gluteal muscle (i) sciatic nerve.

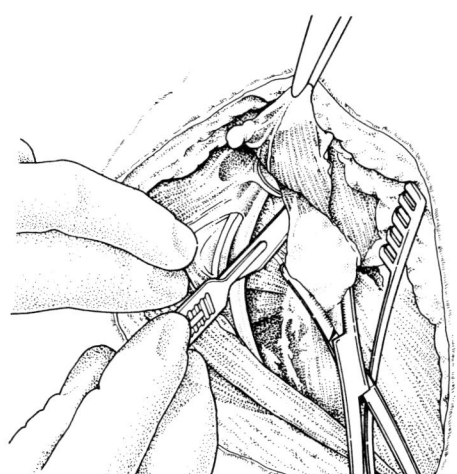

Fig. 7.16. Transection of the obturator and gemelli muscles.

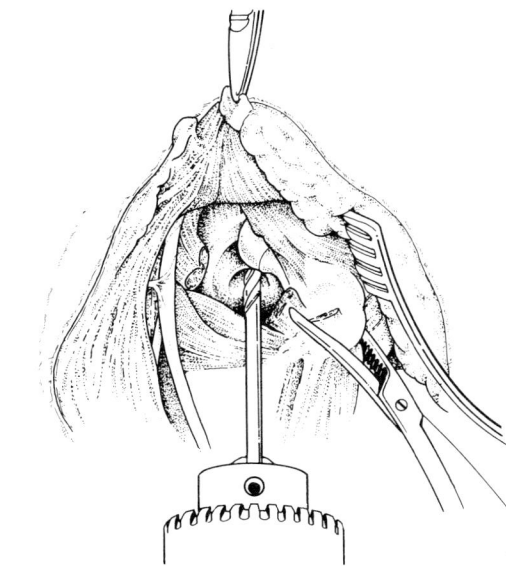

Fig. 7.17. Drilling the acetabulum through the acetabular fossa.

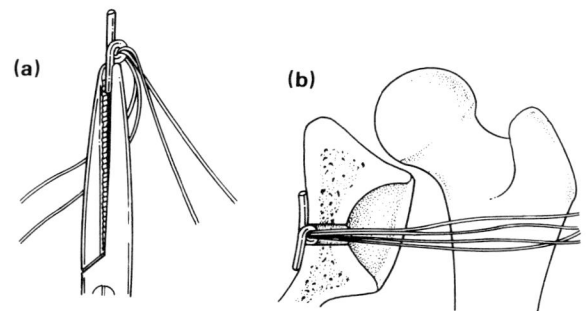

Fig. 7.18. Toggling. (a) Holding the toggle; (b) toggle in position.

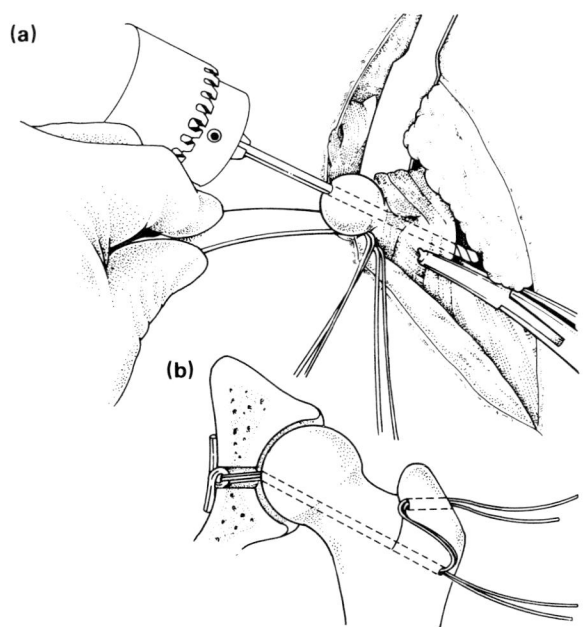

Fig. 7.19. (a) Drilling the femoral head and neck; (b) the great trochanter tunnel.

Arnoczky's 'over the top' procedure for anterior cruciate ligament replacement

Indication

Treatment of the anterior cruciate ligament rupture in dogs over 20 kg bodyweight.

Equipment

A routine surgical set plus a bone chisel (6 mm blade), an orthopaedic hammer, a small hacksaw, a Steinmann pin (4 mm diameter) which is modified as a probe (Fig. 7.21). A 24 gauge wire (monofilament) and braided suture wire on a ½ circle atraumatic type needle.

Technique

The dog is placed on its back for surgery. A skin incision is made over the anterolateral aspect of the stifle to expose the patella and straight patellar ligament. Subcutaneous fat is reflected from these structures. A longitudinal split is made through the medial third of the straight patellar ligament using a scalpel. A parallel incision is also made through the joint capsule on the medial edge of the straight patellar ligament. The two incisions are continued proximally over the medial third of the patella, into the patellar tendon and then in a proximal lateral direction to include a strip of fascia lata (Fig. 7.20). The incisions in the fascia overlying the patella are extended into the bone with a hacksaw. A chisel is then used to elevate a small wedge of bone between the two saw cuts. Care should be taken to avoid penetration of the articular surface of the patella during this procedure. The proximal end of the fascia lata strip, associated patellar tendon with attached patellar wedge and medial third of the straight patellar ligament are now freed to the level of the tibial crest. This strip of tissue from the patella tendon ligament complex is used as a graft to replace the ruptured anterior cruciate ligament.

The existing medial arthrotomy incision is continued proximally and the patella is dislocated laterally (Fig. 7.21). Torn ends of the ruptured anterior cruciate ligament are excised and easily accessible periarticular osteophytes are removed.

The caudal border of the lateral femoral condyle is exposed with the aid of a Hohmann retractor. The blade of the retractor is inserted just proximal to the lateral fabella and used to retract the joint capsule. The tip of the modified Steinmann pin is introduced into the intercondylar fossa and directed along the course of the anterior cruciate ligament. The end of the pin emerges through the caudal joint capsule just proximal to the lateral fabella (Fig. 7.21). The end of a wire loop (24 gauge) is threaded through the hole in the end of the pin, and the pin is withdrawn pulling the loop through the joint (Fig. 7.22). The loop is used to draw the cruciate ligament graft through the joint giving an exact anatomical replacement of the original ligament (Fig. 7.22). The graft is pulled tight, the stifle is flexed to about 35° and the free end of the graft is sutured to the periosteum of the lateral femoral condyle using simple interrupted sutures of multistrand stainless steel wire (Fig. 7.23). The patella is replaced and the medial arthrotomy incision closed with simple interrupted sutures of linen thread or other non-absorbable suture material. Routine wound closure is then carried out.

Postoperative care

A support bandage is applied for a week postoperatively. Antibiotic cover is given for 5 days and skin sutures are removed at 10 days. Exercise is restricted for 4 weeks and then gradually increased.

Although lameness resolves within 3 weeks of surgery in experimental dogs (Arnoczky et al. 1979), in clinical cases the recovery period tends to be longer, 2 months on average. In a postoperative assessment of twenty-eight clinical cases reported by Arnoczky et al. (1979) excellent results were achieved in 61% of cases and good results in 32%.

Complications

1   Penetration of the articular surface of the patella as the cruciate graft is taken might lead to abnormal joint wear and osteoarthritis.
2   Accidental section or breakage of the graft during surgery. When this complication arises it may be possible to repair the graft, an alternative is to use one of the other intra-articular procedures for cruciate replacement, i.e. substitution using fascia lata, skin or braided nylon.
3   The technique restores joint stability immediately and the graft proliferates to approximately three times the original diameter. Therefore a recurrence of joint instability should not be a problem.
4   Persistent lameness following surgery can generally be attributed to pre-existing osteoarthritis.

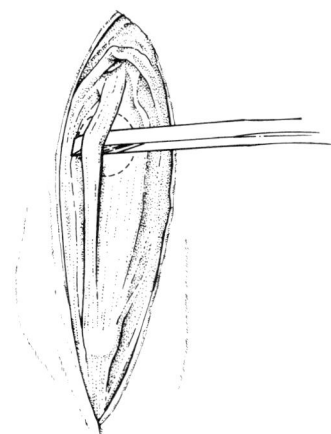

Fig. 7.20. Preparing the strip of straight patellar ligament as the cruciate ligament graft.

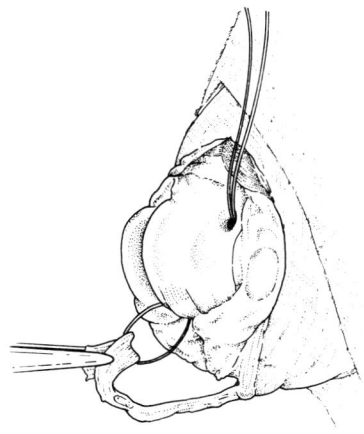

Fig. 7.22. The wire loop in position ready to draw the cruciate ligament graft through the condylar tunnel.

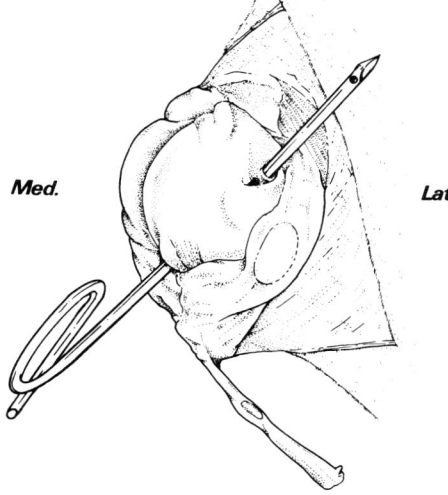

Med. Lat.

Fig. 7.21. Exposure of the femoral condyles. The probe is directed through the joint.

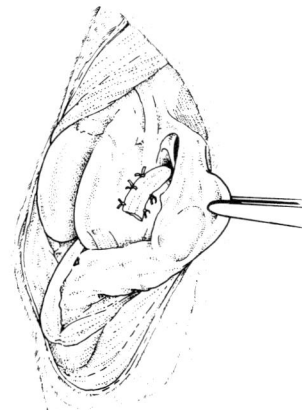

Fig. 7.23. The graft is sutured in position.

Tibial crest transplantation

Indications

Medial luxation of the patella, Grades 2, 3 and 4 (Singleton 1969).
1 Grade 2. Frequent luxation of the patella associated with 15–30° medial deviation of the tibial crest.
2 Grade 3. Permanent medial luxation of the patella associated with 30–60° medial deviation of the tibial crest. The trochlea is usually shallow.
3 Grade 4. Permanent medial luxation of the patella associated with 60–90° medial deviation of the tibial crest. The trochlea is absent or convex.

Equipment

A routine surgical set plus Liston bone-cutting forceps, a Universal bone drill, a straight traumatic needle (to serve as a drill bit), a Hohmann retractor, 24 gauge wire (monofilament), and a Putti type rasp.

Technique

The dog is placed on its back for surgery. A skin incision is made over the anterolateral aspect of the stifle. The joint capsule is incised lateral to the patella and reflected to allow inspection of the trochlea (Fig. 7.24). If the trochlea is shallow or absent, it is deepened. The new groove is carved through the cartilage into the subchondral bone with a scalpel blade and smoothed off with a Putti type rasp (Fig. 7.25). The groove should be large enough to retain the patella and allowance should be made for some infilling which will occur as the defect in the subchondral bone becomes lined by fibrocartilage during healing.

The origin of the anterior tibialis muscle is reflected from the lateral side of the tibial crest. The joint capsule is incised medial to the straight patellar ligament (Fig. 7.24). The blade of a Liston bone-cutting forceps is slid beneath the straight patellar ligament, the blades are closed on either side of the tibial crest and it is cut free proximally but a periosteal attachment is retained distally (Fig. 7.26). The crest is levered laterally with a Hohmann retractor to bring it into line with the trochlea and the patella luxation is reduced (Fig. 7.27).

A tunnel is drilled through the tibial crest and proximal tibia from lateral to medial, using a straight traumatic needle as a drill bit. A length of 24 gauge wire is passed through the tunnel. A second tunnel is drilled from the medial side of the proximal tibia; this does not penetrate the tibial crest but emerges just caudal to it (Fig. 7.28). The medial end of the wire is passed back through this tunnel and the free ends of the wire are twisted tight drawing the tibial crest down firmly in its new lateral position. The medial and lateral arthrotomy incisions are closed next. Excess joint capsule on the lateral side of the patella is overlapped with a double row of sutures while the defect in the medial joint capsule (Fig. 7.27) is covered with a layer of subcutaneous fascia. The anterior tibialis muscle is secured to the straight patella ligament or adjacent joint capsule with mattress sutures. The subcutaneous tissues and skin are closed in routine fashion.

Postoperative care

A support bandage is applied for a week postoperatively. Antibiotic cover is given for 5 days and skin sutures are removed at 10 days. Exercise is restricted for 4 weeks and then gradually increased. In dogs with bilateral patella luxation, a 2 month interval is left between operations on each stifle.

Complications

1 Reluxation of the patella may result from:
(a) Failure to transplant the tibial crest into normal alignment with the trochlea.
(b) Failure to adequately immobilize the tibial crest in its new position.
(c) Failure to provide a trochlea of sufficient depth.
2 Inability to fully extend the stifle joint. This complication is generally seen in dogs with Grade 4 medial luxation when surgical correction has been attempted towards the end of growth or after 1 year of age. Ideally surgical correction should be undertaken at 4–5 months of age, before contracture of the caudal muscles of the stifle has resulted in permanent joint deformity with inability to extend the stifle.

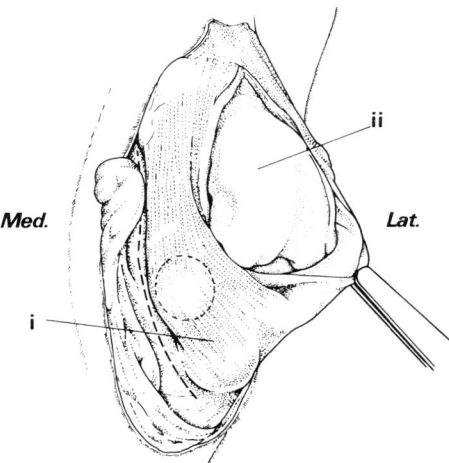

Fig. 7.24. Exposure of the joint. (i) Straight patellar ligament; (ii) femoral condyles.

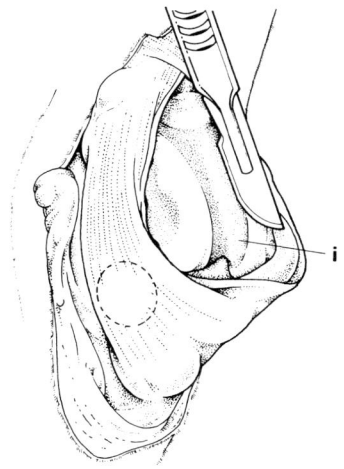

Fig. 7.25. Increasing the depth of the trochlear (i).

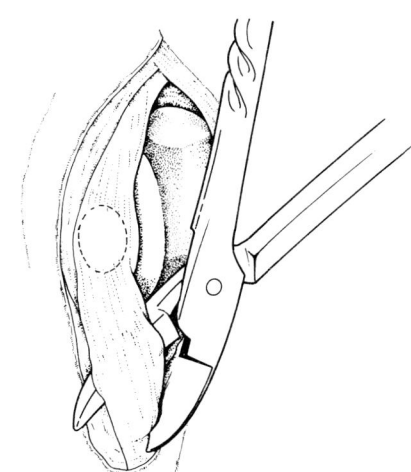

Fig. 7.26. Osteotomy of the tibial crest using the Liston bone cutting forceps.

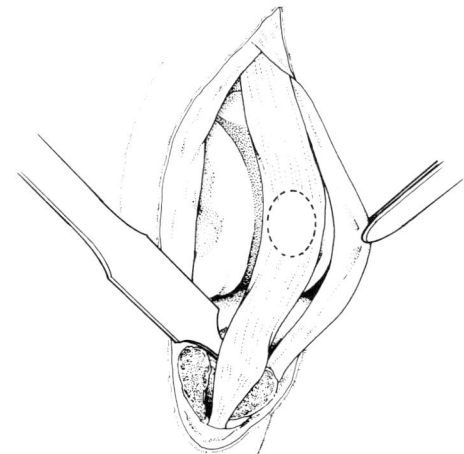

Fig. 7.27. Moving the tibial crest laterally.

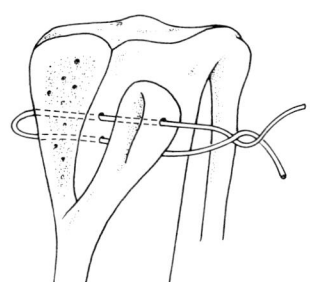

Fig. 7.28. Fixation of the tibial crest.

Chapter 8
Surgery of the Nervous System

JOHN BARKER

Ventral cervical fenestration (Fig. 8.1)

Indications

Surgical indications are intractable pain with poor analgesic response, with or without paresis. Few conditions are more distressing to owner and animal, and early recourse to surgery should be the rule.

Equipment

A routine surgical set, plus fine pointed scalpel and small curved tartar scrapers.

Technique

The dog is anaesthetized, intubated and positioned in dorsal recumbency with the neck arched over a soft sandbag (Fig. 8.2). It is essential to ensure the position is square and stable. The skin incision is from larynx to sternum. Gentle dissection is used to expose the musculature. Division of the sternohyoids is started rostrally and extended caudally to include the sternocephalics. A saline-soaked swab is usually sufficient and controls the minimal bleeding from vessels on the ventral tracheal midline (Fig. 8.3).

The trachea and oesophagus are elevated and their weak attachments cleared with finger and swab, and saline-soaked gauze tape is placed around them and used to displace them away from the operator (Fig. 8.4). The characteristic pattern of the longus colli muscle is revealed (fibres running from the transverse processes of one vertebra to the ventral process on the caudal edge of the body of the next rostral vertebra) and the midline identified. With the animal squarely positioned and adequate exposure, this should cause no problems. Rostrally, the trachea and larynx are more firmly retained in the midline, and slipping a finger beneath here will allow palpation of the sharp ventral process of C1; caudal palpation of sequential ventral processes allows easy identification of the required intervertebral space, which is immediately caudal to the process.

The muscle insertions are cut off two adjacent ventral processes, and a midline incision is made between them (Fig. 8.5). Blunt dissection is then used to separate the muscle and expose the vertebral body, often at surprising depth centrally. The disk appears white and glistening, and insertion of a 25 G hypodermic needle is used to explore the intervertebral space for position and angulation—downwards and rostrally (Fig. 8.5). If any doubt exists of the identification of the disc under exploration, a lateral radiograph can be taken at this point, with the needle *in situ*, without removing the dog from the table. A 'window' is produced in the ventral annulus by two parasagittal incisions, followed by transverse cuts as far rostrally and caudally as possible in the intervertebral space, allowing the 'clean' removal of a portion of annulus (Fig. 8.6a). The upward arching produced by the original positioning of the dog helps at this point. Disc material (resembling toothpaste and chalky white in colour) may well extrude at this point. This is the degenerate and calcified nucleus. A tartar scraper is then used to scoop out remaining material (Fig. 8.6b). The procedure is repeated on any other calcified or protruded disc located radiographically, and as a routine on the first four discs. Statistically, this greatly reduces the chance of the clinical syndrome recurring. Caudal spaces (C6–7, C7–T1) may require the use of an angled tartar scraper to evacuate nuclear material; they are usually operated on only when clear indication of degeneration or protrusion is apparent. Closure is routine, with displaced longus colli muscle being sutured back in the midline with single interrupted catgut stitches, the trachea and oesophagus replaced and the sternohyoid and sternocephalicus sparingly sutured in the midline. A padded neck dressing is applied whilst the dog remains anaesthetized, largely to limit movement as the animal regains consciousness. It is removed within a day or so.

Postoperative care

Routine antibiosis. Cage rest and analgesics are used, with daily clinical reassessment. Most animals are painfree within 48 h, but some, especially if surgery has been delayed, may have some pain for 1 or 2 weeks postoperatively and require continued cage rest. Chronic steroid dosage should not be employed.

Possible complications

Clearance of the ventral muscle off the vertebral body may result in some haemorrhage. This should be rigorously controlled during surgery, both to allow adequate visualization of the operative field and to prevent postoperative haematoma formation. It is impossible at this site to effectively eliminate deadspace.

Postoperative pain may be more apparent if a tentative approach to incising the annulus is taken, and a defined 'window' is not established prior to scooping out the nuclear material.

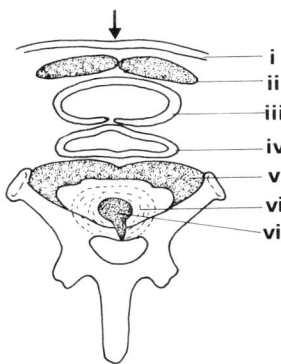

Fig. 8.1. Schematic representation of the area of dissection in ventral cervical fenestration. (i) Skin; (ii) sternohyoid muscles; (iii) trachea; (iv) oesophagus; (v) longus colli muscle; (vi) annulus fibrosus; (vii) nucleus.

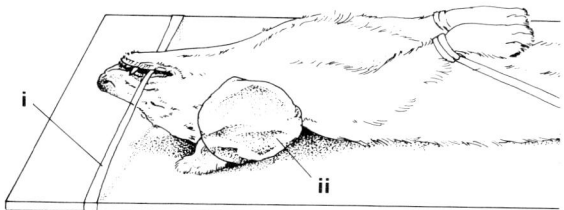

Fig. 8.2. The position for surgery. (i) Restraining tapes; (ii) sandbag to arch the neck.

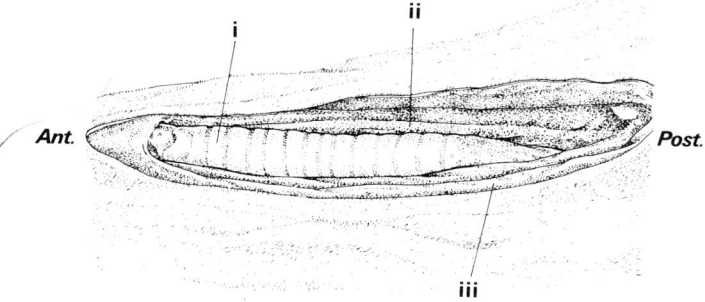

Fig. 8.3. Exposure of the trachea. (i) Trachea; (ii) reflected left sternohyoid muscle; (iii) reflected right sternocephalic muscle.

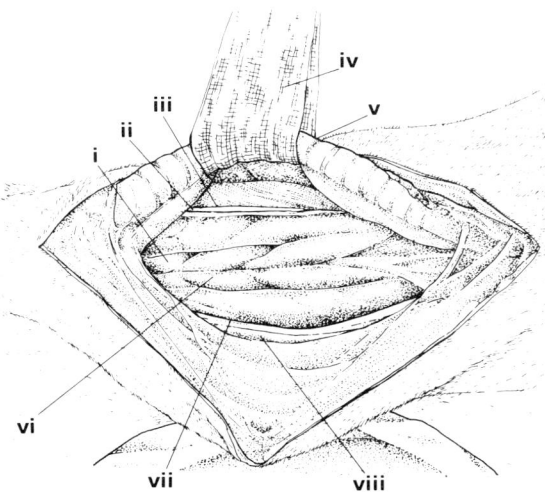

Fig. 8.4. The trachea and oesophagus have been displaced to reveal the longus colli musculature. (i) Ventral vertebral process (palpable); (ii) left vagus nerve; (iii) left carotid artery; (iv) saline soaked tape; (v) trachea; (vi) longus colli musculature; (vii) right vagus nerve: (viii) right carotid artery

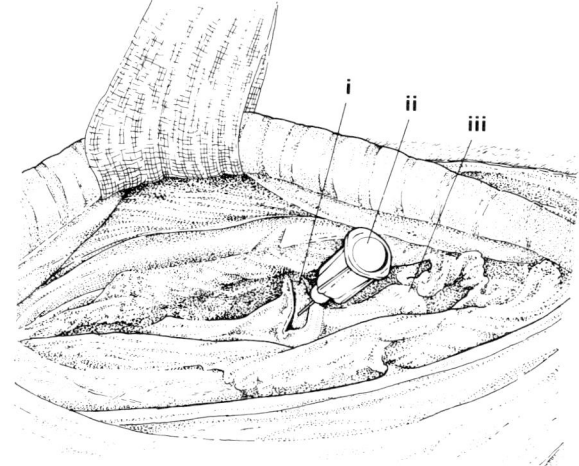

Fig. 8.5. Exposure of the ventral vertebral bodies. (i) Exposed annulus; (ii) 25 G hypodermic needle; (iii) exposed ventral vertebral body.

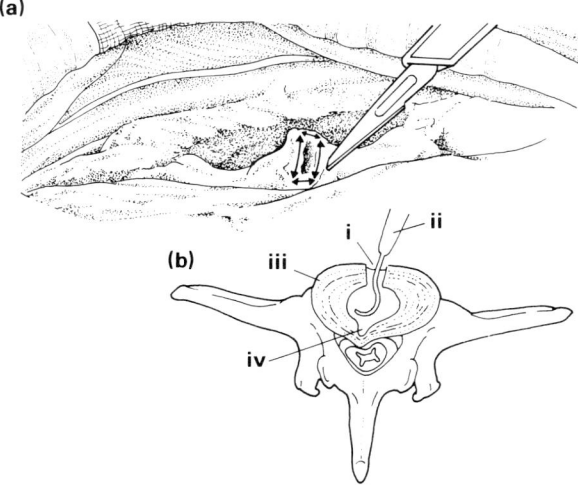

Fig. 8.6. Removal of the disc material. (a) A window is cut in the ventral annulus fibrosus. (b) The tartar scraper being used to scoop out all the disc material, (i) window; (ii) tartar scraper; (iii) annulus fibrosus; (iv) prolapsed nucleus.

Lateral thoracolumbar fenestration

Indications

Cases of thoracolumbar disc protrusion suffering intractable pain, or severe posterior paresis or paralysis with intact hindlimb pain perception and localized neurological signs are suitable for disc fenestration. Animals with no central pain response or signs of extensive cord damage ('ascending spinal syndrome') carry a grim prognosis whatever the treatment. Surgery should be carried out within 24 h if possible.

Equipment

A routine surgical set, plue fine pointed scalpel and small curved tartar scraper.

Technique

The animal is anaesthetized and placed in lateral recumbency (with an inclination maintained by sandbag) with the surface between the dorsal spines and the transverse processes of the thoracolumbar vertebrae directly uppermost (Fig. 8.7). The surgeon then positions himself facing the dog's ventral surface, with its legs towards him. The incision through the skin, subcutaneous fat and dorsal lumbar fascia must be extensive enough to allow for the subsequent retraction of deeper tissue (Fig. 8.8); there is a tendency to incise too far dorsally which must be consciously corrected for. The large iliocostal muscle overlying the transverse processes is identified, and, by palpation of their lateral extremities, the tips of two or more adjacent processes are exposed by incision over them (Fig. 8.8). Muscle is then dissected upwards by periosteal elevation off the dorsal surface of the transverse processes, the established 'plane' of the exposed bone allowing accurate clearing of the muscle between from the intertransverse ligaments (Fig. 8.9). Continued gentle elevation exposes the origin of the process and the rostral, pale (white)

annulus. The segmental nerve and vessels are easily identified, and should be avoided if possible.

The direction and depth of the intervertebral space is determined by the insertion of a 25 G hypodermic needle ventro-medially through the annulus (Fig. 8.10). Degenerate discs frequently show a marked 'bulging' in comparison with their neighbours.

Incision of the annulus is then carried out using a fine-pointed scalpel, making two incisions transversely and two further incisions caudally and rostrally, to remove a square of annulus (Fig. 8.11). A curved fine tartar scraper is then inserted and nuclear material is evacuated by scraping ventrally. The fenestration is carried out on all discs from T/L junction to L5–6 showing calcification of the nucleus, or narrowing of the intervertebral space on radiography. Closure is straightforward, with simple catgut interrupted sutures used to restore displaced tissue.

Postoperative care

Routine antibiosis. A soft body bandage is applied whilst the animal remains anaesthetized. Monitoring recovery comprises daily neurological assessment, combined with cage rest and analgesia. In paraplegic cases, regular (twice daily) attention to bladder emptying and prophylactic broad-spectrum antibiosis (ampicillin), together with attentive nursing, is required. Steroids are not indicated. The bandaging is removed within 3 days.

Possible complications

The most frequently encountered immediate postoperative consequence of surgery is subcutaneous haematoma or seroma formation. Rigorous haemostasis during the procedure with snug bandaging and confinement postoperatively will prevent this. If the procedure is carried out on a paretic patient, tissue handling must be as gentle as possible and great care and patience are required in postoperative nursing to prevent dehiscence, decubital ulceration and/or urinary tract infections.

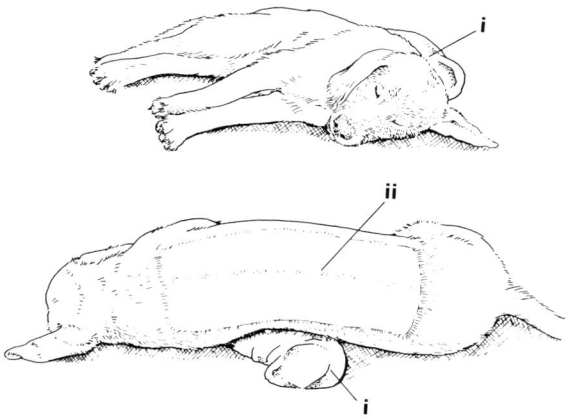

Fig. 8.7. The position for surgery. The surgeon stands facing the ventral body surface. (i) Sandbag; (ii) dorsal midline.

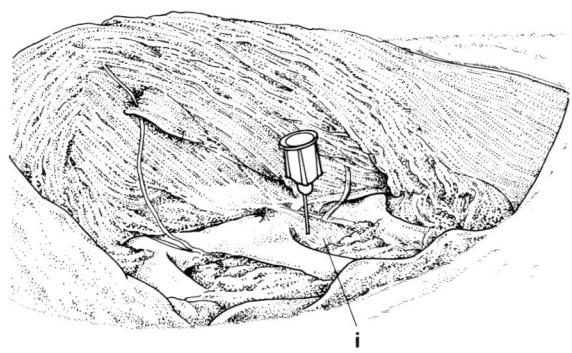

Fig. 8.10. Exploration of the intervertebral space. (i) Annulus fibrosus.

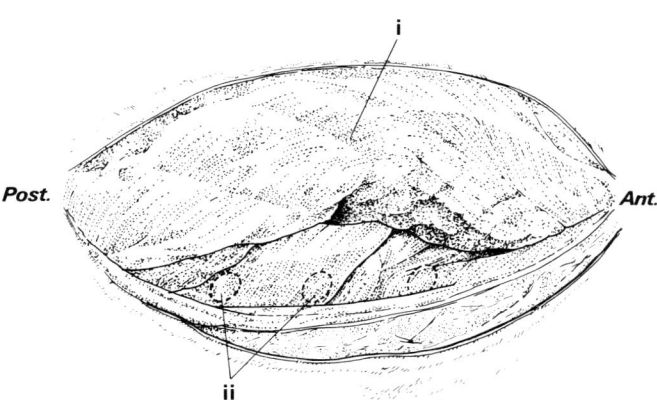

Fig. 8.8. Exposure of the iliocostalis lumborum musculature. (i) Iliocostalis lumborum musculature; (ii) tips of transverse process (palpable).

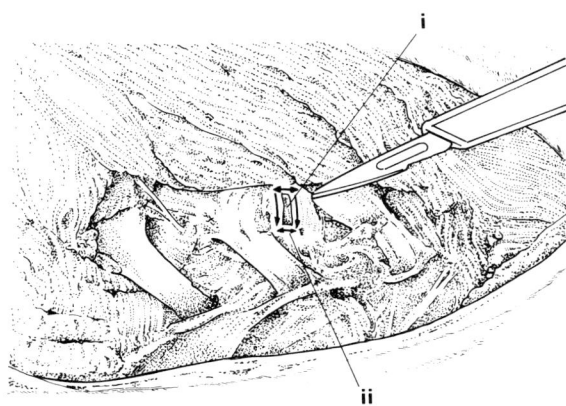

Fig. 8.11. Incision of the annulus fibrosus. (i) Window in the annulus fibrosus; (ii) direction of incision and evacuation (arrows).

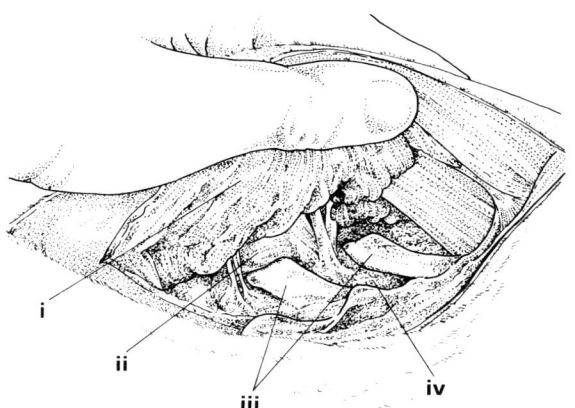

Fig. 8.9. Exposure of the transverse processes. (i) Iliocostalis lumborum musculature; (ii) deep epaxial muscles; (iii) transverse processes; (iv) intertransverse ligament.

The emergency stabilization of spinal fractures or luxations

Indications

The commonest site of damage is at the low thoracic/high lumbar spine. Detailed neurological examination is essential to delineate the extent of cord damage and the prognosis —radiography merely reveals the post-trauma position of the vertebrae. The procedure described enables the practitioner faced with an acute problem to stabilize the site and prevent the animal suffering further cord damage, as a result of its own exertions or of handling by attendents. No specialized equipment or expertise is required, although the technique can be combined with decompressive hemi-laminectomy if desired. Invasion is minimal, and the structures normally maintaining spinal stability are preserved.

Equipment

A routine surgical set, plus Steinmann pins (up to 9/64), 3 G monofilament stainless steel wire, Jacob's chucks, and small drills or Kirschner wires.

Technique

The dog is laid in sternal recumbency, and the initial incision is made midline over the dorsal spines, through skin and subcutaneous fat to expose the fascia over them (Fig. 8.12a). Two parallel incisions are then made to retain a central fascial strip over the supraspinatus ligament, each incision being carried ventro-medially to the lateral surface of the dorsal spines deep to the ligament (Fig. 8.12b). Atraumatic dissection is used to expose the lateral surfaces of the dorsal spines and the articular processes (Fig. 8.13). Muscle attachments to these are cut, and dissection descends into the fossa between them and the base of the dorsal spines to expose the dorsal surface of the arches of two vertebrae either side of the fracture/luxation site.

A Steinmann pin compatible with the animal's size (up to 9/64 can be used) is prebent to around 20° (Fig. 8.14b). A more acute angle precludes insertion. A slightly oversized hole is then drilled in the base of the dorsal spine of the second vertebra, caudal to the fracture/luxation (Fig. 8.14a). The pin is inserted and measured to the middle of the dorsal spine of the second vertebra rostral to the lesion. It is then removed, and one arm (the insertion arm) is cut to this distance. The other is bent inwards at right angles at the measured length and also cut, leaving a small hook equivalent to the thickness of the base of the dorsal spine (Fig. 8.14c). The pin is then reinserted and used to determine the position of the hole to be drilled in the rostral dorsal spine. It is swung out of the way and the hole is drilled exactly sized for the pin (Fig. 8.14a). Single holes are drilled through the intervening dorsal spines using Kirschner wire and 3 G monofilament stainless steel wire inserted (Fig. 8.15). The pin is positioned as shown with the wire in figure-of-eight loops around it and is bent under tension into its final position and held there whilst the wire loops are tightened to retain it (Fig. 8.16 and Fig. 8.17).

The muscle is then replaced, and the fascia sutured to the central strip. Skin closure is routine, and a padded body bandage is applied before recovery from anaesthesia to aid in maintaining stability as consciousness returns.

Postoperative care

Routine antibiosis. The dog is cage rested and subjected to serial neurological examination and assessment.

Possible complications

This technique involves considerable tissue handling and blunt dissection, coupled with the insertion of an extensive prosthesis—conditions which lend themselves to wound infection and dehiscence. Pre- and postoperative antibiosis and gentle handling are essential. Haemostasis should be rigorous throughout to avoid haematoma formation.

In young dogs, the dorsal spines are easily fractured. The unconscious patient must be handled with great care postoperatively, and the provision of temporary external padded support is sensible.

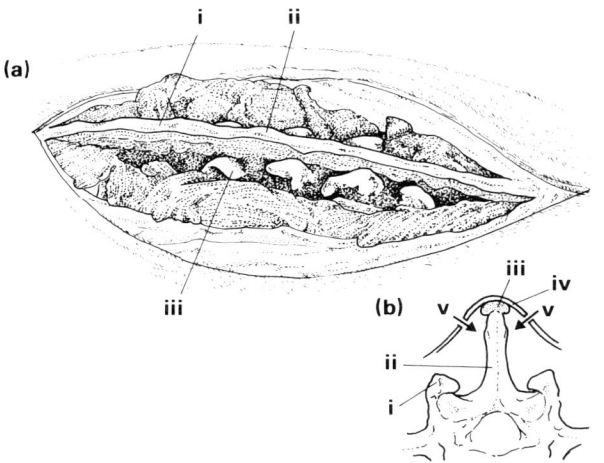

Fig. 8.12. Exposure of the dorsal spine. (a) The midline skin incision, (i) central fascial strip; (ii) dorsal spines; (iii) articular processes. (b) Exposure of the lateral surfaces of the spines, (i) articular process; (ii) dorsal spines; (iii) supraspinatus ligament; (iv) central fascial strip; (v) incisions.

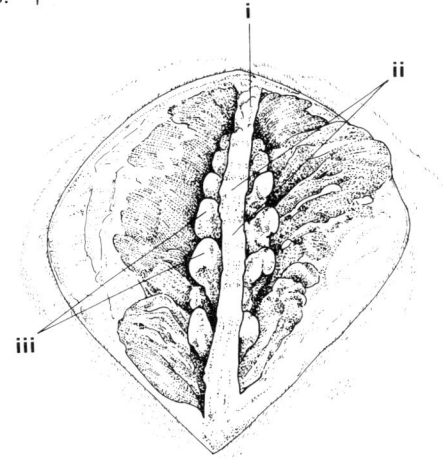

Fig. 8.13. Exposure of the lateral surfaces of the spines. (a) Central fascia strip; (b) dorsal spines; (c) articular processes.

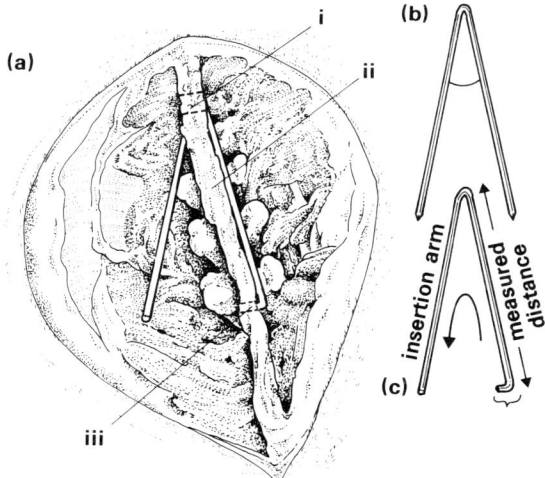

Fig. 8.14. The use of the Steinmann pin. (a) The position (i) of drill holes posterior to the lesion; (ii) position of the lesion; (iii) position of the drill hole anterior to the lesion. (b) Steinmann pin bent at 20°. (c) Pin cut and finally shaped.

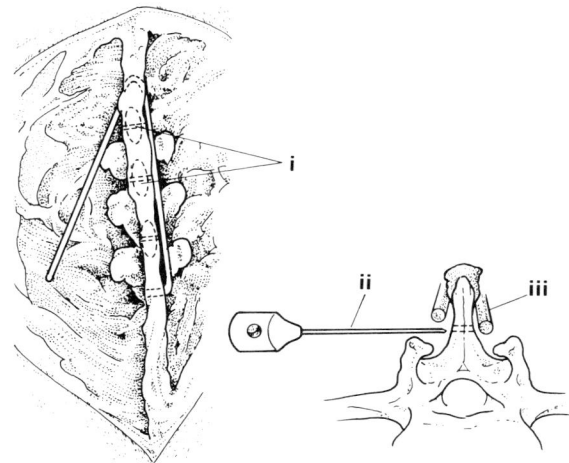

Fig. 8.15. Insertion of the Steinmann pin. (i) Position of the fine drill holes; (ii) Kirschner wire; (iii) pin.

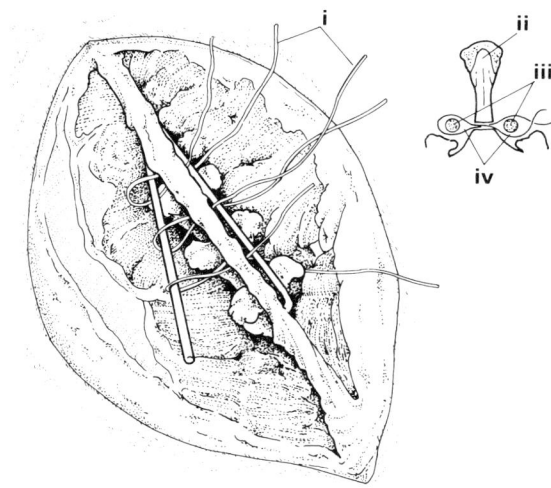

Fig. 8.16. Pin fixation using the monofilament stainless steel wire. (i) 3 G monofilament wire; (ii) dorsal spine; (iii) Steinmann pin; (iv) wire figure-of-eight.

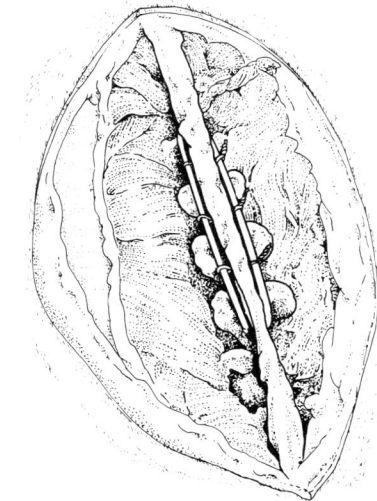

Fig. 8.17. The pin *in situ* prior to closure.

Emergency peripheral nerve surgery

Indications

The practitioner must be ready to carry out peripheral nerve repair within 8 h of injury if the best possible outcome for the animal is to be achieved in cases arising from iatrogenic nerve severance, as complication of limb fracture or from severe trauma. In infected post-traumatic wounds, the concern is for primary repair to allow successful later (21 day) exploration and surgery, possibly in a referral clinic.

Equipment

Fine (ophthalmic) forceps, scissors, needleholders (dry heat sterilized), 7-0 silk with attached cutting needle. Gloves, swabs, drapes and instruments must be detritus free (talc, lint, etc.).

Technique

Any 'landmarks', for example the pattern of nerve fibre bundles in cut ends, cross-sectional shape of nerve, presence of small blood vessels, must be identified to allow accurate anastomosis, without longitudinal twisting (Fig. 8.18). There must be no tension of the anastomosis suture line. The nerve should be elevated from the underlying tissue and dissected free for a considerable length either side of the discontinuity (Fig. 8.19). The tough but almost transparent epineurium is the only portion gripped by for-

ceps or pierced by needle point. Minimal sutures are used to anchor the two portions to underlying fascia or muscle in the same tissue plane, and to ensure that the two cut ends are opposed without tension (Fig. 8.20a). Minimal single interrupted sutures are then used to anastomose them accurately, using the 'landmarks' described (Fig. 8.20b). All sutures should be laid before tying and, when tying, any excessive twist in the suture material should be relieved. Clotted plasma (from centrifuged autogenous blood) is used to close the anastomosis site (Fig. 8.20c). Surrounding tissues are restored as simply as possible, avoiding tension or distortion, and external support is given where indicated.

Postoperative care

Routine antibiosis.

Possible complications

Although the procedure as described is intended as an emergency primary repair, failure to maintain strict asepsis, atraumatic tissue handling and exclusion of detritus from the operative field will preclude later success. Haemostasis must be absolute. Any breakdown in technique will lead to excess scarring and prevent secondary exploration.

Postoperatively, the use of massage and passive exercise will prevent muscle atrophy and loss of limb function. The remotest chance of self-mutilation of the denervated area must never be allowed to arise.

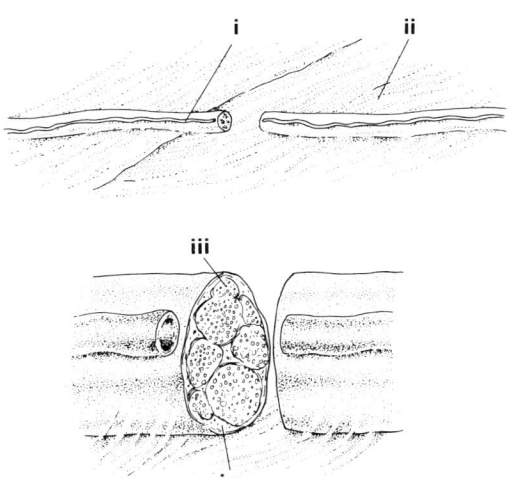

Fig. 8.18. Identification of landmarks. (i) Small blood vessel; (ii) fascia, muscle; (iii) pattern of fibre bundles; (iv) epineurium.

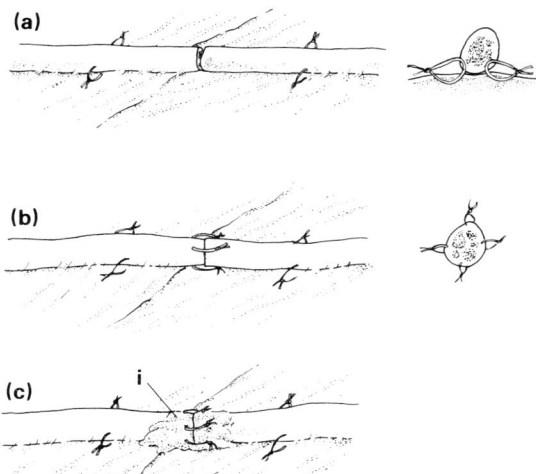

Fig. 8.20. The suturing technique. (a) The placement of the 'anchor' sutures; (b) anastomosis (minimal suture material); (c) sealing the anastomosis site with clotted plasma (i).

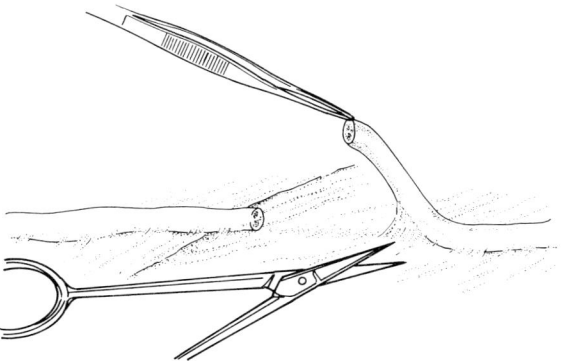

Fig. 8.19. Elevation and mobilization of the nerve.

Suggested Further Reading

Section 1

Surgical instrumentation

Bellenger C.R. (1982) Sutures I. The purpose of sutures and available suture materials. *The Compendium of Continuing Education.* **4**, 507.

Bellenger C.R. (1982) Sutures II. The use of sutures and alternative methods of closure. *The Compendium of Continuing Education.* **4**, 587.

Hurov L. (1978) *Handbook of Veterinary Surgical Instruments and Glossary of Surgical Terms.* W.B. Saunders Co, Philadelphia.

Knecht C.D., Allen A.R., Williams D.J. & Johnson J.H. (1981) *Fundamental Techniques in Veterinary Surgery.* 2nd ed. W.B. Saunders Co, Philadelphia.

Markowitz J., Archibald J. & Downie H.G. (1964) *Experimental Surgery.* 5th ed. Williams & Wilkins, Baltimore.

Miller M.E., Allgöwer M., Schneider R. & Willenegger H. (1979) *Manual of Internal Fixation.* 2nd ed. Springer-Verlag, Berlin.

Anaesthesia and fluid therapy

Dorsch S.A. & Dorsch S.E. (1977) *Understanding Anaesthesia Equipment.* Williams & Wilkins Co., Baltimore.

Hall L.W. & Clarke K. (1983) *Veterinary Anaesthesia*, 8th ed. Bailliere Tindall, London.

Lumb W.V. & Jones E.W. (1973) *Veterinary Anaesthesia.* Lea & Febiger, Philadelphia.

Sawyer D.C. (1982) *The Practice of Small Animal Anaesthesia.* W.B. Saunders Co, Philadelphia.

Soma L.R. (1971) *Textbook of Veterinary Anaesthesia.* Williams & Wilkins Co., Baltimore.

Radiography

Douglas S.W. & Williamson H.D. (1980) *Principles of Veterinary Radiography*, 3rd ed. Bailliere Tindall, London.

Morgan J.P., Silverman S. & Zontine W.J. (1977) *Techniques of Veterinary Radiography.* Veterinary Radiology Associates, Davis, California.

Ryan G.D. (1981) *Radiographic Positioning of Small Animals.* Lea & Febiger, Philadelphia.

Ticer J.W. (1984) *Radiographic Technique in Veterinary Practice*, 2nd ed. W.B. Saunders Co, Philadelphia.

Webbon P.M. (1981) *Guide to Diagnostic Radiography in Small Animal Practice.* BSAVA, London.

Section 2

Chapter 1: The repair of the skin

Archibald J. (1974) *Canine Surgery*, 2nd ed. American Veterinary Publications Inc., Santa Barbara.

Archibald J. (in press) *Canine and Feline Surgery*, 3rd ed. American Veterinary Publications Inc., Santa Barbara.

Bojrab M.J. (1981) *A Handbook on Veterinary Wound Management.* The Kendall Co., Boston.

Converse J.M. (1977) *Reconstructive Plastic Surgery: General Principles, vol. 1*, 2nd ed. W.B. Saunders Co., Philadelphia.

Pavletic M.M. (1983) Plastic and reconstructive surgery in the dog and cat. In: Bojrab M.J. (ed.). *Current Techniques in Small Animal Surgery*, 2nd ed. Lea & Febiger, Philadelphia.

Peacock E.E. Jr. (1984) *Wound Repair*, 2nd ed. W.B. Saunders Co, Philadelphia.

Swaim S.F. (1978) Management and reconstruction of traumatized skin. *Vet. Audio Review*, **7**.

Swaim S.F. (1980) *Surgery of Traumatized Skin. Management and Reconstruction in the Dog and Cat.* W.B. Saunders Co, Philadelphia.

Swaim S.F. (1982) Reconstruction of problem skin defects of the head, neck and trunk. *Sci. Proc. 49th Ann. Amer. Anim. Hosp. Assoc. Mtg.*, 1982.

Chapter 2: Surgery of the head and neck region

Bedford P.G.C. (1984) Ear, nose, mouth and throat. In: Chandler E.A. *et al.* (eds). *Canine Medicine and Therapeutics.* Blackwell Scientific Publications, Oxford.

Bojrab M.J. (1975) *Current Techniques in Small Animal Surgery.* Lea & Febiger, Philadelphia.

Böhning R.H., De Hoff W.D., McElhinney A. & Hofstra P.C. (1970) Pharyngostomy for maintenance of the anorectic animal. *J. Amer. Vet. Med. Assoc.* **156**, 611.

Cawley A.J. & Archibald J. (1974) *Plastic Surgery in Canine Surgery.* American Veterinary Medical Publications, Santa Barbara.

Rosin E. & Hanlon G.F. (1972) Canine cricopharyngeal achalasia. *J. Am. Vet. Med. Assoc.* **160**, 1496.

Rubin G.J., Neal T.M. & Bojrab M.J. (1973) Surgical reconstruction for collapsed tracheal rings. *J. Small Anim. Pract.* **14**, 607.

Spreull J.S.A. (1963) Surgery of the nasal cavity of the dog and cat. *Vet. Rec.* **75**, 105.

Spreull J.S.A. & Head K.W. (1967) Cervical salivary cysts in the dog. *J. Small Anim. Pract.* **8**, 17.

Chapter 3: Thoracic surgery

Archibald J. & Harvey C.E. (1974) *Canine Surgery*, 2nd ed. American Veterinary Publications Inc., Santa Barbara.

Brasmer T.H. (1975) In: Bojrab, M.J. (ed.). *Current Techniques in Small Animal Surgery*, 2nd ed. Lea & Febiger, Philadelphia.

Ettinger S.J. & Suter P.F. (1970) *Canine Cardiology.* W.B. Saunders Co, Philadelphia.

Kagan K.G. (1980) *Veterinary Clinics of North America: Trauma.* W.B. Saunders Co, Philadelphia.

Chapter 4: Surgery of the abdominal alimentary tract

Betts C.W., Wingfield W.E. & Rosin E. (1976) 'Permanent' gastropexy—as a prophylactic measure against gastric volvulus. *J. Am. Anim. Hosp. Ass.* **12**, 177.

Dann J.R. (1976) Medical and surgical treatment of canine acute gastric dilatation. *J. Am. Anim. Hosp. Ass.* **12**, 17.

Dingwell J.S. & Eger C.E. (1976) Management of acute gastric dilatation with torsion and rupture: a case report. *J. Am. Anim. Hosp. Ass.* **12**, 23.

Douglas S.W., Hall L.W. & Walker R.G. (1970) The surgical relief of gastric lesions in the dog—Report of seven cases. *Vet. Rec.* **86**, 743.

Funkquist B. (1979) Gastric torsion in the dog III. Fundic gastropexy as a relapse-preventing procedure. *J. Small Anim. Pract.* **20**, 103.

Funkquist B. & Garmer L. (1967) Pathogenetic and therapeutic aspects of torsion of the canine stomach. *J. Small Anim. Pract.* **8**, 523.

Funkquist B. & Obel N. (1979) Gastric torsion in the dog II. Nonsurgical treatment by aspiration of gastric contents during repeated rotation of the animal. *J. Small Anim. Pract.* **20**, 93.

Parks J.L. & Greene R.W. (1976) Tube gastrostomy for the treatment of gastric volvulus. *J. Am. Anim. Hosp. Ass.* **12**, 168.

Pass M.A. & Johnston D.E. (1973) Treatment of gastric dilation and torsion in the dog: gastric decompression by gastrostomy under local analgesia. *J. Small Anim. Pract.* **14**, 131.

Ravitch M.M. (1979) Intussusception in infants and children. In Najarian J.S. & Delaney J.P. (eds.) *Gastrointestinal Surgery*. U.S.A. Symposia Specialists Inc., Florida.

Walshaw R. & Johnston D.E. (1976) Treatment of gastric dilatation—volvulus by gastric decompression and patient stabilization before major surgery. *J. Am. Anim. Hosp. Ass.* **12**, 162.

Weaver A.D. (1977) Canine intestinal intussusception. *Vet. Rec.* **100**, 524.

Williams D.A. & Burrows C.F. (1981) Short bowel syndrome—a case report in a dog and discussion of the pathophysiology of bowel resection. *J. Small Anim. Pract.* **22**, 263.

Chapter 5: Surgery of the urino-genital tract

Annis J.R. & Allen A.R. (1967) *An Atlas of Canine Surgery*. Lea & Febiger, Philadelphia.

Archibald J. & Harvey C.E. (1974) *Canine Surgery*, 2nd ed. American Veterinary Publications Inc., Santa Barbara.

Bojrab M.J. (1975) *Current Techniques in Small Animal Surgery*. Lea & Febiger, Philadelphia.

Leonard E.P. (1968) *Fundamentals of Small Animal Surgery*. W.B. Saunders Co., Philadelphia.

Chapter 6: Ocular surgery

Bistner S.I., Aguirre G. & Batik G. (1977) *Atlas of Veterinary Ophthalmic Surgery*. W.B. Saunders Co., Philadelphia.

Gelatt K.N. (1982) *Veterinary Ophthalmology*. Lea & Febiger, Philadelphia.

Chapter 7: Orthopaedic surgery

Arnoczky S.P., Tarvin G.B., Marshall J.L. & Saltzman B. (1979) The 'over the top' procedure: a technique for anterior cruciate ligament substitution in the dog. *J. Am. An. Hosp. Ass.* **15**, 283.

Denny H.R. & Gibbs C. (1980) The surgical treatment of osteochondritis dissecans and ununited coronoid process in the canine elbow. *J. Small Anim. Pract.* **21**, 323.

Grøndalen J. & Rørvik A.M. (1980) Arthrosis in the elbow joint of young rapidly growing dogs IV. Ununited anconeal process. *Nord. Vet. Med.* **32**, 212.

Knowles A.T., Knowles J.O. & Knowles R.P. (1953) An operation to preserve the continuity of the hip joint. *J. Am. Vet. Med. Ass.* **123**, 508.

Olsson S.E. (1975) Lameness in the dog. *Proc. Am. Anim. Hosp. Ann. Meet.* 42–363.

Singleton W.B. (1969) Stifle deformities in the dog. *J. Small Anim. Pract.* **10**, 59.

Vaughan L.C. & Jones D.G.C. (1968) Osteochondritis dissecans of the head of the humerus in dogs. *J. Small Anim. Pract.* **9**, 283.

Chapter 8: Surgery of the nervous system

Braund K.G. *et al.* (1976) Lateral spinal decompression in the dog. *J. Small Anim. Pract.* **17**, 583.

Denny H.R. (1978) The surgical treatment of cervical disk protrusions in the dog: A review of 40 cases. *J. Small Anim. Pract.* **19**, 251.

Denny H.R. (1978) The lateral fenestration of canine thoracolumbar disk protrusions: A review of 30 cases. *J. Small Anim. Pract.* **19**, 259.

Funkquist B. (1978) Investigations of the therapeutic and prophylactic effects of disk evacuation in cases of thoracolumbar herniated disks in dogs. *Acta. vet. scand.* **19**, 441.

Funkquist B. & Svalastoga E. (1979) A simplified approach to the last two cervical disks of the dog. *J. Small Anim. Pract.* **20**, 593.

Gage E.D. (1971) Surgical repair of spinal fractures in small-breed dogs. *V.M./S.A.C.* **66**, 1095.

Swaim S.F. (1975) Thoracolumbar and sacral spine trauma. In: Bojrab M.J. (ed.). *Current Techniques in Small Animal Surgery I*. Lea & Febiger, Philadelphia.

Swaim S.F. (1975) Isolated peripheral nerves. In: Bojrab M.J. (ed.). *Current Techniques in Small Animal Surgery I*. Lea & Febiger, Philadelphia.

Yturraspe D.J. & Lumb W.V. (1972) The use of plastic spinal plates for internal fixation of the canine spine. *J. Am. Vet. Med. Ass.* **161**, 1651.

Index